Phenomenology and nursing research

Michael Crotty

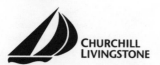

CHURCHILL LIVINGSTONE

CHURCHILL LIVINGSTONE
An imprint of Pearson Professional (Australia) Pty Ltd

Kings Gardens
95 Coventry Street
South Melbourne VIC 3205
Australia

Pearson Professional offices in Hong Kong, Singapore, Japan, USA, Canada, India,
United Kingdom and Europe.

First published 1996

National Library of Australia
Cataloguing-in-Publication data

   Crotty, Michael,
   Phenomenology and nursing research.

   Bibliography.
   Includes index.
   ISBN 0 443 05432 0.
   1. Nursing - Research. 2. Phenomenology. I. Title.

610.73072

Edited by Trischa Baker
Produced by Churchill Livingstone in Melbourne
Printed in Australia

Contents

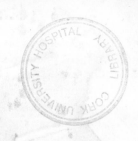

Preface

I am very much in phenomenology's debt.

More than thirty years ago, existential phenomenology played a pivotal role in liberating me, and several close colleagues of the time, from shackles forged by the grandest of grand theories. Mediated by the writings of contemporary European thinkers — Dutch, Belgian, French and German authors, for the most part — phenomenology offered us an approach that drew its starting point from authentic experience and insisted that we return to authentic experience at every point along our way.

This book has been written in the firm conviction that, several decades on and in a quite different world, phenomenology of that kind still has relevance and usefulness. I hope my readers find it so.

Oppression takes many forms and is incarnate in the very language we speak and write. As far as the oppression of women is concerned, a number of authors quoted in these pages wrote at a time when there was little, if any, consciousness of this. They blithely talk of 'man' when they mean women and men, and feel free to use the generic masculine whenever they need pronouns. My readers will readily recognise such usages, and no doubt deplore them, as they occur in the quotations given. There is hardly need for me to interrupt the text *ad nauseam* by inserting '(*sic*)' many times over to point them out.

It is to a woman that I dedicate this book. I thank my wife, Christina, for her encouragement and help. Her ability to stay close to her own immediate experience of the world and to prize it for what it is worth has always seemed to me unaffected phenomenology-in-action.

The book is dedicated also to my three teenaged children. For some time now, they have been the only members of their respective classes who have known how to pronounce and spell the word 'phenomenology'. For this they appear singularly unthankful and vow they never want to hear the word again. *Si jeunesse savait, si vieillesse pouvait ...*

Michael Crotty

The physicist's atoms will always appear more real than the historical and qualitative face of the world, the physico-chemical processes more real than the organic forms, the psychological atoms of empiricism more real than perceived phenomena, the intellectual atoms represented by the 'significations' of the Vienna Circle more real than consciousness, as long as the attempt is made to build up the shape of the world (life, perception, mind) instead of recognizing, as the source that stares us in the face and as the ultimate court of appeal in our knowledge of these things, our *experience* of them.

It is that as yet dumb experience ... which we are concerned to lead to the pure expression of its own meaning

Maurice Merleau-Ponty

No higher court for the individual exists than meanings or self-interpretations embedded in language, skills, and practices. No laws, structures, or mechanisms offer higher explanatory principles or greater predictive power than self-interpretations in the form of common meanings, personal concerns, and cultural practices shaped by a particular history. The goal is to understand everyday practices and the experiences of health and illness.

Experience then is considered the active history of a tradition that can be captured in narratives of the practice.

Patricia Benner

Introduction

In social research today, at least in the English-speaking world, there are two phenomenologies.

One of them is the phenomenology of the phenomenological movement spawned by Edmund Husserl. Describing that as 'one' phenomenology is not to deny the broadness and diversity of this movement. Among its many vagaries, it stretches from the transcendental phenomenology of its founder to the existential phenomenology espoused and expounded by thinkers such as Sartre, Merleau-Ponty, Ortega y Gasset, Marcel and Ricoeur. In many cases, and in many respects, the figures historically associated with the phenomenological movement make strange bedfellows. If one can speak at all of an orthodoxy in this tradition, it has to be said that, right from the start, there has been an abundance of heretics.

Nevertheless, while phenomenologists of this tradition prove a most diverse group, they continue to share a basic approach. There is a common core to their understanding and their method of inquiry. As the respected historian of the phenomenological movement Herbert Spiegelberg insists, even if there are as many phenomenologies as there are phenomenologists, there *needs* to be such a common core if the use of the common label is to be justified.[1]

That common core is not to be found in the other phenomenology. Its mode of understanding and its method of inquiry are very different. It is an approach to social inquiry that has sprung up particularly in the last three decades or so, and it is very much a North American development. Originally, American thinkers were slow to give any kind of acceptance, let alone welcome, to this strange European philosophy and its offshoot developments in fields such as psychology and sociology. Certainly, the work of Alfred Schutz led to phenomenology having significant impact in American sociology. Schutz, at least in his later work, was himself influenced by the American intellectual tradition, and this was even more true of those who followed Schutz down phenomenological pathways within sociology. In the end, the indigenous line of thought well and truly prevailed. In the field of psychology, almost from the start, the impact of the American tradition was nothing less than overwhelming. While there have been and are North American psychologists engaged in genuinely phenomenological endeavours, they have been relatively few in number. In the 1960s, American-style humanistic psychology was already at centre stage when phenomenologists like van Kaam and Giorgi began articulating their stepwise methods for phenomenological research. What seems to have happened is that while the rhetoric of phenomenology proved attractive, the phenomenological method itself was interpreted in the light of prevailing concepts and became fundamentally distorted.

It could be said that in being transplanted to the North American continent, phenomenology experienced significant mutations. Transplantation may not be the analogy to use. For the most part, rather than being permitted to set down its own roots west of the Atlantic, phenomenology was grafted on to local stock. The fruit it has produced reflects the American intellectual tradition far more than any features of its parent plant. True enough, the discourse of phenomenology remains. The vocabulary is there. One hears of 'experience' and 'phenomenon', of 'reduction' and 'bracketing' — of 'intentionality', even. However, the meaning of these terms is no longer the meaning they have borne within the phenomenological movement from which they have been taken.

This kind of phenomenology is informed by, or at least is perfectly compatible with, the very epistemological stance which traditional phenomenology seeks to refute. Quite clearly, what we are seeing now is a *new* phenomenology and it will be referred to as such in this work.

A line of thought that is new and different is to be welcomed. It should not be rejected because it is new. Nor, in this case particularly, can one complain that it is laying claim to a name which is already spoken for. While the term 'phenomenology' is generally taken today to refer to the movement stemming from Husserl, it was used in many different senses before Husserl and even now is used by people in different ways.

So what is wrong with a new approach emerging and calling itself phenomenology, even if it differs radically from the standard version? Is there any problem in that? Yes, there is. In fact, there seem to be two problems. The first is the failure of the new phenomenologists to recognise the newness of what they are doing. The second is more serious: their failure to recognise the value of what they are not doing.

It would seem important, on grounds of basic scholarship if nothing else, that people espousing a new phenomenology should recognise its newness. It is doubtful that they do. In expounding their approach, they are found routinely to cite authors like Husserl, Merleau-Ponty or Schutz as if these thinkers were involved in an enterprise that in some way resembles their own. The new phenomenologists, it appears, consider themselves in continuity with the mainstream phenomeno-logical movement.

A much more important consideration is the loss incurred when the understanding and approach inherent in mainstream phenomenology are bypassed, as they clearly are in the new phenomenology. This second problem stems from the first. Because the exponents of the new phenomenology believe they are doing authentic phenomenology, they are satisfied that what phenomenology has to offer is already in their hands. Consequently, they no longer look to original sources or even to contemporary representatives of the phenomenological movement. This, it may be suggested, is impoverishing.

Impoverishing in what way? What is lost by an exclusive adherence to the new phenomenology? What would be regained through a return to a more authentic phenomenology? The answer may be summed up in two words: *objectivity* and *critique*.

Those familiar with the new phenomenology have heard its oft-repeated claim: it seeks to establish the subjective experience of the people it studies. The new phenomenologists have meticulously developed step-by-step methods of inquiry and analysis whose paramount purpose is precisely to preserve the subjective character of their data intact and untainted.

As we shall see, mainstream phenomenology does not share this kind of subjectivism. It is a study of phenomena, i.e. of the *objects* of human experience. It elucidates *what* people experience. If it inquires into how certain subjects experience this or that, it is not for the sake of learning and describing how these particular people feel, perceive and understand. The new phenomenology does have that kind of focus and the research it inspires may seek, for example, to describe how its subjects feel ('Did these people feel ashamed?'). Mainstream phenomenological research has a different scope. It aims to illuminate, precisely as human phenomena, the feelings that people experience ('What is shame as a phenomenon that people experience?'). The new phenomenology works hard at gathering people's subjective meanings, the sense they make of things ('What does giving post-mortem nursing care mean to these nurses?'). Mainstream phenomenology, in contrast, wants to elucidate, first and foremost, the phenomena to which people are attaching meaning. It pursues, not the sense people make of things, but what they are making sense of ('What is post-mortem nursing care as a phenomenon that nurses experience *before* they make any sense of it?'). In Eugene Kaelin's phrase, phenomenology is 'a trip back to the facts of our perceptive experience'.[2] Hence phenomenology's traditional slogan: 'Back to the things themselves!'

True enough, the 'things themselves' prove elusive. In describing what comes into view within immediate experience, we draw on language and therefore on culture. These are tools we have to employ. For that reason, we end, not with a presuppositionless description of phenomena, but with

3

re-interpretation. This will be as much a construction as the sense we have laid aside, but as re-interpretation — as new meaning or renewed meaning — it is precisely what we as phenomenologists are after.

This orientation to the object means, among other things, that mainstream phenomenology is not subjectivistic and individualistic, as the new phenomenology tends to be. The charge of excessive individualism has long been levelled at various forms of traditional American thought. As many see it, this individualism reached new heights with the emergence of humanistic psychology. Humanistic psychology seems to have played a key role in informing the new phenomenology. Other strands of American pragmatism and social analysis have played their part too. These influences, not the phenomenological tradition, have shaped what tends to present itself as phenomenology in the English-speaking world today.

This self-styled phenomenology shares the subjectivism for which humanistic psychology is so often criticised. Excessive subjectivism becomes a narcissism. Christopher Lasch has written of the 'culture of narcissism',[3] while, according to Rollo May,[4] the narcissistic personality described by Lasch is 'a further development of American individualism' and narcissism constitutes 'the neurosis of our time'. Narcissism may seem too strong a word to use in describing the new phenomenology. If so, it may be somewhat less provocative to talk of its overwhelming subjectivism. A turn to mainstream phenomenological perspectives could serve as a counter to this type and degree of subjectivism, for it would introduce a much-needed note of objectivity into our discussion of human reality.

A phenomenology more in tune with that of the tradition would not only be more objective; it would also be more *critical*. The phenomenology of the phenomenological movement is a thoroughly critical methodology. 'Phenomenological philosophy is first of all philosophical criticism', writes Richard Zaner.[5] Phenomenology calls upon us to lay aside for the moment — to 'bracket' — our everyday perceptions and accepted understandings so as to encounter afresh that to which we are attributing meaning. In this way it calls into question meanings that we take for granted. In this 'laying aside' and this 'calling into question', nothing is sacred. Armstrong puts it quite strongly:

> Phenomenology is much more than a suspension of assumptions. The phenomenological reduction is a change of attitude that throws suspicion on everyday experiences.[6]

What phenomenology requires is a radical attempt to return to pre-reflective, pre-predicative experience — to our experience as it is immediately given to us *before* we make sense of it. This means a return to the possibilities for meaning which our experience offers. As Sadler, an existential phenomenologist, expresses it:

Our experience is no less than an existential encounter with a world which has a potentially infinite horizon. This human world is not predetermined, as common sense or physicalist language would indicate; it is a world that is open for the discovery and creation of ever-new directions for encounter, and hence open to the emergence of as yet undiscovered significance. Because our experience is a creative and thoroughly historical encounter in a lived world, one that is alive with our encounter of it, it is potentially open to new possibilities of significant existence.[7]

In talking of suspending our meanings and going back to that primordial 'something' we made sense of in the first place, we are not speaking in terms of individual chronology. After all, when we reflect on life experience, our own or anyone else's, we know that, for the most part, it has not been a matter of encountering phenomena and making sense of them one by one. Instead, we are born into a whole world of meaning. We are taught meanings. We have bestowed upon us a comprehensive system of significant symbols.

We are essentially cultural creatures. It is culture that makes us human. So our culture — our symbols, our meaning systems — is to be seen as liberating. It allows us to emerge from our immediate environment and to reflect upon it. It offers us the possibility of knowing our past and planning our future. This freedom-bestowing, ennobling, enriching, symbol-bearing culture is what the symbolic interactionist explores *par excellence*. The symbolic interactionist is caught up in a profound fascination with our enculturated ways of knowing, understanding and communicating.

The phenomenologist's interest is otherwise. The goal of phenomenological inquiry goes beyond identifying, appreciating and explaining current and shared meanings. It seeks to critique these meanings. It does this by suspending them so as to initiate a long, hard look at the objects of immediate experience to which they are attributed.

In this, phenomenologists have no argument at all with what symbolic interactionists or similarly minded social investigators accept or do. Nevertheless, in agreeing that culture is liberating, phenomenologists remain very aware that it is also limiting. While it sets us free, it also sets boundaries. Culture may make us human, but it does so in a quite definite and circumscribing way — in and through *this* particular culture, *this* special system of significant symbols, *these* meanings. In imposing these meanings, it is excluding others.

There is more than that. Our symbol system is not only limited and limiting. It is also a barrier. It not only stands *for* things but comes to stand *between* things and us — more precisely, between us and our immediate experience of objects. In other words, it tends to exclude or at least inhibit the immediate experience of what we make sense of through it. It tends to substitute itself for what we actually see, hear, feel, smell, taste or even imagine.

Phenomenology is about putting that meaning system in abeyance. Far from inviting us to explore our everyday meanings as they stand, it calls upon us to lay them aside for the moment and to open ourselves to the phenomena in their stark immediacy to see what emerges for us. In Merleau-Ponty's terms, this would be a 'direct and primitive contact with the world',[8] engendering 'another kind of thought, that which grasps its object as it comes into being'.[9] For decades now Kurt Wolff has been presenting this notion as 'surrender-and-catch'. Wolff invites us to surrender to the phenomenon and then, like those fishing in the sea, to lift our net and see what we have caught.[10] Merleau-Ponty uses the same metaphor:

> Husserl's essences are destined to bring back all the living relationships of experience, as the fisherman's net draws up from the depths of the ocean quivering fish and seaweed.[11]

What we will have caught may be new meaning. Or it may be old meaning that has had new life breathed into it, for it will no longer be meaning we have merely inherited or borrowed but *our* meaning, begotten authentically from our very own experience. It is transformed by the process. Natanson describes for us the nature and outcome of this phenomenological process:

> ... 'already-given' objects are newly displayed in the theater of consciousness. The consequence of that display is the propagation of meaning, the enlargement of experience.[12]

The contrast between the laying aside of everyday meaning in phenomenology and the exploration of everyday meaning in a pragmatist, symbolic-interactionist approach is obvious. The pointing up of the contrast here is not meant to be pejorative. The contrast in no way detracts from the undeniable merit of that other line of thought. Pragmatism and its offshoots constitute a rich intellectual tradition and Eugene Rochberg-Halton's claim that pragmatism 'speaks to the contemporary hunger for significance'[13] is more than justified. The pragmatism and symbolic interactionism referred to here are not pragmatism and symbolic interactionism in their origins and their high points but more popularised versions of pragmatist and interactionist approaches to be found in sociology textbooks and manuals of research methodology. To accuse Charles Sanders Peirce, William James, John Dewey or George Herbert Mead of being either individualistic or acritical is surely to engage in caricature.[14]

Individualistic? We need only recall how Dewey, for his part, took issue with the individualism which he claimed had entered the picture — as a 'distortion' — with 'the modern discovery of inner experience'.

Failure to recognise that this world of inner experience is dependent upon an extension of language which is a social product and operation led to the subjectivistic, solipsistic, and egotistic strain in modern thought.[15]

Acritical? Take Peirce as an example. Peirce was not one to rest content with exploring the cultural complex of his time and place. For him, '*pragmatism* is not a *Weltanschauung* but it is a method of reflexion having for its purpose to render ideas clear.'[16] As it happens, Peirce developed his own version of phenomenology — 'phaneroscopy' he came to call it in the end — independently of Husserl. As he strove to determine the elemental categories present to the mind in their 'Firstness' or qualitative immediacy, Peirce was engaged on a task that closely resembles the phenomenologists' efforts to delineate phenomena encountered in immediate experience.[17]

In short, between the pragmatist tradition at its best and the phenomenological movement at its best there is much in common. There is enough in common for them to engage with each other in fertile fashion and produce something that is both genuinely new and eminently worthwhile. If that had happened, one could have nothing but applause for both the process and the outcome. But that did not happen. The new phenomenology adds little, if anything, to what the symbolic interactionism of the textbooks and humanistic psychology already had to offer. And what they had to offer was essentially illustrative rather than critical.

So something *is* lost when one is content to accept the new phenomenology and looks no longer to mainstream phenomenology. That so-called phenomenology simply describes the state of affairs instead of problematising it. It looks to what is taken for granted but fails to call it into question: on the contrary, it perpetuates traditional meanings and reinforces current understandings. It remains preoccupied with 'what is' rather than striving, however laboriously and tentatively, towards 'what might be'. At best, this entails a failure to capture new meanings and a loss of opportunities for revivifying the understandings that possess us. At worst, it allows oppression, exploitation and unfreedom to persist without question.

Yes, there are two phenomenologies — and they are far apart. This book attempts to outline what each of them is and what the differences are. As far as the new phenomenology is concerned, our picture of what it is about will be drawn from the field of nursing research. Nurse researchers yield to none in the warmth with which they have embraced this approach.

More than this, in the firm conviction that a more genuinely phenomenological mode of social inquiry serves important purposes, the book comes in the end to detail a method for engaging in precisely that sort of inquiry. In this respect, it is more than an invitation to reflection. It is an invitation also to research and action.

NOTES

1 See Spiegelberg (1982), p. 677.
2 Kaelin (1965), p. 38.
3 See Lasch (1979).
4 May (1991), pp. 112–14.
5 Zaner (1970), p. 79.
6 Armstrong (1976), p. 252.
7 Sadler (1969), p. 20.
8 Merleau-Ponty (1962), p. vii.
9 *Ibid.*, p. 120.
10 See Wolff (1972, 1976, 1983, 1984, 1989a, 1989b, 1990). Wolff more than once emphasises the differences between his surrender-and-catch and the phenomenology of Husserl, but there is no doubt that his approach squares with what Spiegelberg posits as the essential elements and the 'common core' of true phenomenology.
11 Merleau-Ponty (1962), p. xv.
12 Natanson (1985), p. 12.
13 Rochberg-Halton (1986), p. ix.
14 Not everyone would agree with this statement. Lewis Mumford, for example, describes the pragmatism of James and Dewey as an 'attitude of compromise and accommodation' (1950, p. 49). Social critic Randolph Bourne, himself a pragmatist and an associate of Dewey, deplores the uncritical character he sees pragmatism assuming in his contemporaries, including his erstwhile mentor. He wants pragmatism's openness, optimism and progressivism to be tested 'inch by inch'. It is not enough, Bourne claims, merely to clarify the values we hold. We 'must rage and struggle until new values come out of the travail' (1977, p. 345). While these seem to be overly harsh judgements as far as James and Dewey are concerned, they are surely warranted when applied to the forms of pragmatism that came to prevail.
15 Dewey (1925), p.173.
16 Peirce (1931–58), Vol.5, p. 9.
17 See Spiegelberg (1981a).

1

The case of nursing research

Even a cursory glance at nursing research literature reveals the popularity of the 'phenomenological approach'. Ask your friendly librarian for the latest CINAHL CD-ROM disk and select the articles that show 'phenomenology' among the descriptors. You can expect a listing that contains several hundred titles.

It may be true, as Anderson claims,[1] that a 'review of articles in nursing journals over the past decade shows that some scholars are moving not only away from logical positivism but beyond phenomenology and hermeneutics'. If so, those moving beyond phenomenology seem to have no trouble in having their places filled.

What do the nurse researchers who espouse the 'phenomenological method' consider phenomenology to be? In attempting to answer that question, there are many paths one might follow. For better or worse, the method adopted here has been to take published nursing research that claims to be phenomenological and subject this to close examination and analysis. For this purpose, thirty pieces of such research[2] have been chosen at random.[3] Hopefully, these are representative of the thinking of nurse researchers more generally. The fact that significantly new information seemed to dry up long before the thirtieth article is somewhat reassuring in this respect.

The articles fall into two categories. Most simply talk about 'phenomenology' and the 'phenomenological method' and, if they refer at all to the origin of their phenomenology, they cite Edmund Husserl. Five articles[4] expressly claim to be Heideggerian in approach and for that reason merit special consideration.

At this point all thirty articles are taken together and the question is put again: what is the picture of phenomenology that emerges from them?

The thirty pieces of published nursing research examined in this book

Anderson, J M (1991a). 'Immigrant women speak of chronic illness: the social construction of the devalued self'. *Journal of Advanced Nursing* 16:6 (June), pp. 710–717.

Beck, C T (1991a). 'How students perceive faculty caring: A phenomenological study'. *Nurse Educator* 16:5 (September–October), pp. 18–22.

Beck, C T (1991b). 'Undergraduate nursing students' lived experience of health: a phenomenological study'. *Journal of Nursing Education* 30:8 (October), pp. 371–374.

Beck, C T (1992). 'The lived experience of postpartum depression: a phenomenological study'. *Nursing Research* 41:3 (May–June), pp. 166–170.

Bennett, L (1991). 'Adolescent girls' experience of witnessing marital violence: a phenomenological study'. *Journal of Advanced Nursing* 16:4 (April), pp. 431–438.

Bowman, J M (1991). 'The meaning of chronic low back pain'. *AAOHN Journal* 39:8 (August), pp. 381–384.

Breault, A J and Polifroni, E C (1992). 'Caring for people with AIDS: nurses' attitudes and feelings'. *Journal of Advanced Nursing* 17:1 (January), pp. 21–27.

Diekelmann, N L (1992). 'Learning-as-testing: a Heideggerian hermeneutical analysis of the lived experiences of students and teachers in nursing'. *Advances in Nursing Science* 14:3 (March), pp. 72–83.

Dobbie, B J (1991). 'Women's mid-life experience: an evolving consciousness of self and children'. *Journal of Advanced Nursing* 16:7 (July), pp. 825–831.

Elfert, H, Anderson, J M and Lai, M (1991). 'Parents' perceptions of children with chronic illness: a study of immigrant Chinese families'. *Journal of Pediatric Nursing* 6:2 (April), pp. 114–120.

Eyres, S J, Loustau, A and Ersek, M (1992). 'Ways of knowing among beginning students in nursing'. *Journal of Nursing Education* 31:4 (April), pp. 175–180.

Hauck, M R (1991). 'Mothers' descriptions of the toilet-training process: a phenomenologic study'. *Journal of Pediatric Nursing* 6:2 (April), pp. 80–86.

Henderson, A D and Brouse, A J (1991). 'The experiences of new fathers during the first three weeks of life'. *Journal of Advanced Nursing* 16:3 (March), pp. 293–298.

Keefe, M R and Froese-Fretz, A (1991). 'Living with an irritable infant: maternal perspectives'. *MCN* 16:5 (September–October), pp. 255–259.

Lethbridge, D J (1991). 'Choosing and using contraception: toward a theory of women's contraceptive self-care'. *Nursing Research* 40:5 (September–October), pp. 276–280.

Marr, J (1991). 'The experience of living with Parkinson's disease'. *Journal of Neuroscience Nursing* 23:5 (October), pp. 325–329.

Martin, L S (1991). 'Using Watson's theory to explore the dimensions of adult polycystic kidney disease'. *ANNA Journal* 18:5 (October), pp. 493–496.

Mason, C (1992). 'Non-attendance at out-patient clinics: a case study'. *Journal of Advanced Nursing* 17:5 (May), pp. 554–560.

McHaffie, H E (1991). 'Neonatal intensive care units: visiting policies for grandparents'. *Midwifery* 7 (September), pp. 122–132.

Monahan, R S (1992). 'Nursing home employment: the nurse's aide's perspective'. *Journal of Gerontological Nursing* 18:2 (February), pp. 13–16.

Montbriand, M J and Laing, G P (1991). 'Alternative health care as control strategy'. *Journal of Advanced Nursing* 16:3 (March), pp. 325–332.

Newman, M A and Moch, S D (1991). 'Life patterns of persons with coronary heart disease'. *Nursing Science Quarterly* 4:4 (Winter), pp. 161–167.

Rather, M L (1992). '"Nursing as a way of thinking": Heideggerian hermeneutical analysis of the lived experience of the returning RN'. *Research in Nursing and Health* 15:1 (February), pp. 47–55.

Rose, J F (1990). 'Psychologic health of women: A phenomenologic study of women's inner strength'. *Advances in Nursing Science* 12:2 (January), pp. 56–70.

Watson, P (1991). 'Care or control: questions and answers for psychiatric nursing practice'. *Nursing Praxis in New Zealand* 6:2 (March), pp. 10–14.

Whetstone, W R and Reid, J C (1991). 'Health promotion of older adults: perceived barriers'. *Journal of Advanced Nursing* 16 (November), pp. 1343–1349.

Wolf, Z R (1991). 'Nurses' experiences giving postmortem care to patients who have donated organs: a phenomenological study'. *Scholarly Inquiry for Nursing Practice: An International Journal* 5:2 (Summer), pp. 73–87.

Wondolowski, C and Davis, D K (1991). 'The lived experience of health in the oldest old: a phenomenological study'. *Nursing Science Quarterly* 4:3 (Fall), pp. 113–118.

Wood, F G (1991). 'The meaning of caregiving'. *Rehabilitation Nursing* 16:4 (July–August), pp.195–198.

Zerwekh, J V (1992). 'Laying the groundwork for family self-help: locating families, building trust, and building strength'. *Public Health Nursing* 9:1 (March), pp. 15–21.

Phenomenology: A study of experience

Most of the researchers cited here leave no doubt that they consider phenomenology to be about 'experience'. Twenty-five of them indicate this expressly.[5]

They also have a lot to say about the *kind* of experience they are referring to.

First of all, to use a word beloved of phenomenologists generally, they are clearly speaking of 'mundane' experience. Not that our authors use this word. They refer instead to 'lived' experience[6] or experience 'as lived',[7] to 'everyday' or 'day-to-day' experience,[8] to 'human' experience or experience 'as humanly lived',[9] to 'existential' experience or experience 'as it exists'.[10]

On the face of it, it may not seem fair to lump these expressions together and take them all to be referring to 'mundane' or 'everyday' understanding of experience. After all, at least some of these terms have the potential to denote a special class of experiences. In some hands, terms such as 'lived experience' and 'existential experience' stand for prereflective or prepredicative experience, i.e. experience before it is reflected on or thought about. It is clear, however, that this is not the kind of experience that these researchers are focusing on. For example:

- Anderson says she is inquiring into 'the existential experience of chronic illness by immigrant women'. Nevertheless, in the exemplary case history she presents, her data are said to come from a 'narrative account' giving us the informant's 'construction of the illness experience' and showing 'how she made sense of these experiences'.
- Breault and Polifroni invoke 'lived experience' but identify it with 'the perspective of the nurse'.
- 'The aim of phenomenology', explain Elfert, Anderson and Lai (in terms drawn from Oiler), 'is to describe experience as it is lived by people.' Still citing Oiler, they go on to refer to 'lived experience'. Does 'lived experience' or 'experience as it is lived by people' mean something different from everyday experiences understood in everyday terms? It is clear that, for these authors, it does not. 'Researchers who use this perspective', say Elfert and her associates, 'aim to understand the subjective meaning of everyday life experiences from the perspective of the informants.'

There is one exception and this will be discussed in Chapter 3. That case apart, these nurse researchers have their sights firmly set on everyday understandings of everyday experiences.

Secondly, as has already emerged, our authors are talking of experience peculiar to the individuals concerned. It is, many of them say,[11] experience as understood from the individuals' 'perspective', 'frame of reference' or 'point of view', i.e. 'participants' experience as they see it'. Yes, it is 'subjective' experience,[12] 'personal' experience, with significance for people 'personally'.[13] What is looked for is 'first person description'.[14]

Given such strong emphasis on the individuality of experience, it is somewhat perplexing to find that, when they come to analyse their data, the interest of most of these researchers tends to focus exclusively on 'themes' and 'shared experience' — in short, on commonalities rather than what is peculiar to the individual. For example:

- 'In the discipline of phenomenology,' Montbriand and Laing insist, 'it is the task of the researcher to gain entry into the conceptual world of the informants, allowing them to construct and give meaning to their own reality.' Nevertheless, the aim they present for their study is to 'recreate for the reader the shared beliefs, practices, artifacts, folk knowledge, and behaviours of some groups of people'.
- Marr recognises the individuality of personal experience ('Although the subjects' general experiences were quite similar, each subject's personal experience was unique'), but she also informs her readers that 'analysis of individual interviews did not occur in isolation; rather, all data were analyzed together in their entirety'.
- Bennett wants access to the phenomenon 'exactly as it reveals itself to the experiencing subject in all its concreteness and particularity' (she is citing Giorgi here), but she ends with a 'general-level description' synthesised from 'shared themes and meanings'. This expresses for her the 'essential structure' of the marital violence that forms the focus for her study.

Here we find an express search for individual, subjective meanings curiously linked to a method that systematically discards individual, subjective meanings unless they are shared with other respondents. There is an anomaly here and it is encountered repeatedly within the new phenomenology.

If phenomenology centres on people's individual, everyday experience, how does it relate to that experience? The researchers point to a multi-faceted relationship.

At the very least, phenomenology serves to *highlight* the realm of experience. It 'affirms subjective experience'.[15] Its methods 'emphasize the importance of the subjective experience'.[16] Accordingly, the phenomenological approach places the 'focus of attention'[17] on our experiences and we are encouraged to 'return'[18] to them. They are to be identified[19] and studied[20] and the context in which they are embedded is to be examined.[21]

The purpose of studying experiences is to understand them — their nature, their meaning, their essential structure.[22] A phenomenological method will 'uncover meaning' and provide 'hermeneutical interpretation of the meaning of human experience in its situated context'.[23] In short, phenomenology seeks 'to render lived experience intelligible'.[24]

Because it provides such understanding, the phenomenological approach permits description of experience.[25] More than that, it actually provides description[26] — even 'exhaustive description'[27] — of experience and its meaning and structure.

In this way the researchers make it crystal clear that, as they see it, phenomenology is about addressing, identifying, describing, understanding and interpreting the experiences people have in their day-to-day lives and precisely *as* those people have the experiences and understand them.

What the researchers fail to make clear is the meaning they are attributing to the word 'experience'. None of them offer a definition or explanation of it. The reader must work that out from the general content of the article. This is not usually a difficult task. According to Breault and Polifroni, for instance, their study 'was conducted to identify the feelings and attitudes that nurses associate with caring for people with AIDS'.[28] They also state that the study employed the phenomenological approach in 'an attempt to identify and describe the experience of caring for PWAs'.[29] It seems legitimate to conclude that, for Breault and Polifroni, 'experience' is to be understood as people's feelings and attitudes.

Working in this fashion, it is possible to identify six understandings of the word 'experience' in this collection of articles:

- feelings or emotional states[30]
- perceptions, meanings[31]
- perceptions, attitudes, feelings (a combination of the two preceding understandings)[32]
- events[33]
- events, together with personal reactions to events (a combination of the two preceding understandings)[34]
- function or role (such as nursing, schooling or caregiving).[35]

It is also possible to identify that the pivotal notions are 'feelings', 'attitudes' and 'meanings' (or 'perceptions'). Even where the word 'experience' does not immediately encompass them, these notions clearly constitute the focal point of the writers' interest.

Phenomenology: The study of phenomena

This multiplicity of meanings of 'experience' is compounded by confusion regarding the meaning of 'phenomena'.

Ten of the articles[36] associate phenomenology with the study of phenomena. Since this is the etymological meaning of the word, the fact that only one-third pay attention to phenomena is somewhat surprising. Those who do refer to phenomena feel no need to define the term — which is also surprising because it has had a critical, if rather ambiguous, history within the phenomenological movement. Still, our authors have a number of things to say *about* phenomena.

We are told, for instance, that phenomena are both 'humanly'[37] and 'consciously'[38] experienced. This would seem to confirm the everyday use of the word to denote 'what is experienced', i.e. the object of experience.

Phenomena are described by the subjects[39] and studied by the researcher.[40] Indeed, the goal of phenomenology is to 'gain access to the phenomenon',[41] study 'phenomena on their own ground',[42] achieve 'experiential understanding' and 'full elaboration' of the phenomenon,[43] and make its meaning or essence clear.[44]

To succeed in this enterprise, one must be 'open to the phenomenon' and remain 'faithful to the phenomenon as a whole'.[45]

Much of this is reminiscent of the language used about 'experience' and raises the question whether, and in what way, 'experience' and 'phenomenon' are to be distinguished. Our authors prove to be less than helpful in this respect, even though the question has central importance in determining what phenomenology is about.

For a start, there appears to be a difference of opinion among the authors. Are we seeking to learn about phenomena through descriptions of experiences (as Bowman, Marr and Wolf assert, for example) or to understand experiences through the study of phenomena (as Henderson and Brouse, together with Beck, are claiming)?

According to Bowman, it is the phenomenon that is experienced and, if we can obtain descriptions of experiences and analyse them, we will uncover the phenomenon's meaning.

> The phenomenological method 'seeks to uncover the meaning of humanly experienced phenomena through the analysis of subjects' descriptions' (Parse) ... In the phenomenological method individuals are asked to describe experiences ...[46]

Marr and Wolf agree: we learn about phenomena and their meaning through 'personal'[47] or 'subjective'[48] experience.

Beck muddies the waters. She claims the opposite: we learn of experience via knowledge of phenomena, not the other way round.

> Discovery of the meaning of human experiences through the analysis of subjects' written or oral descriptions of phenomena is the purpose of phenomenology.[49]

Henderson and Brouse are saying much the same sort of thing, at least if events in one's life are taken as phenomena. These researchers are concerned with the experiences of new fathers, i.e. during the first three weeks after the birth of their child.

> In order to uncover the meanings that experiences held for these fathers, a phenomenological method was used. This method allowed us to understand client experiences by analysing events in their lives ... The researcher attempts to understand the client's reality and the context in which this reality exists ...

Phenomenology, with its focus on 'the unfolding of the phenomenon itself [to] guide the logic of the inquiry' (Giorgi 1975), emphasizes the importance of the researcher understanding the meaning that people's experiences hold for them.[50]

It would seem that Beck, along with Henderson and Brouse, is saying the opposite of what Bowman, Marr and Wolf are claiming. But does Beck really mean it? Her study seeks 'to answer the question: What is the essential structure of a caring nursing student–faculty interaction?' She asks students to describe what they regard as 'caring' situations, expressing their 'thoughts, perceptions and feelings'. The outcome for Beck is the understanding that caring, as the students perceive it, involves:

- an attentive presence
- a sharing of selves
- a number of consequences, such as a sense of being respected and valued, an urge to reach out to others, and a feeling of being energised and rejuvenated.

This seems to be an attempt to use described experiences to develop an understanding of the 'phenomenon' of caring interaction rather than the other way round. The method Beck adopts for data analysis is said to culminate in an 'exhaustive description of the investigated phenomenon'. In another study, she arrives at 'three necessary constituents of the phenomenon of health'.[51] Beck, then, may not be doing what she claims to be doing.

Nor are Henderson and Brouse, when one comes to look at their research attentively. They take account of events in the fathers' lives and they appear to regard events as 'phenomena'. But how do they gain knowledge of the experiences they come to describe? The experiences in question are the 'intense emotions' felt by the fathers because of conflicting information prior to the birth, their distress that they and their spouses were unable to be supportive to each other, their expectations before the birth, their reactions when reality began to intrude after the birth, and their sense of comfort as they began to feel more in charge of things. The researchers' knowledge of these experiences comes from a direct description of the experiences by the fathers, not from any 'unfolding of the phenomenon' or 'analysing events in their lives'. These writers, too, are not doing what they claim to be doing.

Perhaps, to cross to the other side of the fence, the same can be said of Wolf. The outcome of Wolf's research is an 'exhaustive description of the postmortem experiences of nurses'. Wolf claims that we learn of phenomena through people's subjective experiences and hopes that the exhaustive description 'will explicate the nature of these subjective experiences and delineate the essence of the phenomenon'. What does she mean by 'essence of the phenomenon'? The method adopted for data analysis leads to an identification of the 'essential structure of the postmortem care experience'. Moreover, the section towards the end of Wolf's article headed 'Essential structure' turns out to be a summary of the perceptions, attitudes, feelings and practices associated with post-mortem care by nurses. It makes sense to speak of post-mortem nursing care as a phenomenon. It is, after all, an object of nurses' experience. In that case, it must be said that Wolf's study begins with phenomenon and ends with subjective experiences — the contrary of what Wolf claims to be doing.

Marr too appears to be saying one thing and doing another. She tells her readers:

> Since the purpose of the study was to explore a lived experience, the phenomenological method was used to describe the experience of living with PD. The major assumption of this approach is knowledge about particular phenomena is best obtained by tapping subjects' personal experiences.[52]

According to Marr, then, exploring the lived experience, i.e. tapping the personal experiences of the subjects, will provide knowledge of the phenomenon. All well and good, but in the end Marr is content to claim that her study 'represents an initial step toward understanding the subjective experience of living with Parkinson's disease'.

There would appear to be much confusion of thought here regarding the nature and relationship of 'experience' and 'phenomenon'. Indeed, despite talk of seeking one through the other, for most of these researchers they are clearly interchangeable terms. For instance, Anderson puts in parallel 'narrative accounts of the experience of illness' and 'the phenomena described by women in the in-depth interviews'. In talking of 'phenomena on their own ground', Elfert and her co-researchers show that they mean 'the subjective meaning of everyday life experiences from the perspective of the informants'. Rose tells us that her interviews 'continued until the participants felt that they had finished or exhausted their descriptions of the phenomenon'. What she had asked each participant to describe was 'her lived experience of inner strength — her feelings, thoughts and perceptions'.[53] It would appear from this that one's feelings, thoughts and perceptions about the phenomenon *are* the phenomenon. Wolf, as we have seen, also puts the two together: she hopes that her 'exhaustive description of the postmortem experiences of nurses will explicate the nature of these subjective experiences and delineate the essence of the phenomenon'.[54] Add to this the fact that, while Giorgi is cited in Henderson and Brouse to the effect that phenomenological inquiry is guided by the unfolding of the *phenomenon*, for Bowman (and Omery whom she is quoting) Giorgi's method of analysis lets the *experience* unfold 'as it exists for the subject'. Omery herself clearly identifies 'phenomenon 'and 'experience'. 'The goal of the phenomenological method', she tells her readers, 'is an accurate description of the experience or phenomenon under study.'[55]

While these nurse researchers seem on the whole to be using 'phenomenon' and 'experience' interchangeably, there is a hint in some of them that the phenomenon is the essence or central meaning of the experience. Linked to this is the notion, found in several of these authors, that the phenomenon is what emerges when the researcher puts the essential elements of the experience together. Take Bennett, for example. She 'seeks to gain access to the phenomenon', but what she does in the end is to 'synthesize' seven core themes so as to express a 'general level description' of what was experienced. It seems that, for Bennett, phenomenon means a synthesis of the main elements of the experience. Dobbie may be viewing things in much the same light. She wants 'to ensure accuracy and full elaboration of the phenomenon'. The word 'elaboration' suggests that, for her too, the phenomenon is what emerges when the central elements of the experience are put together. Something similar can be found in Rather, for whom 'incorporating the contributions of all persons involved in the analytic process' is the way 'to further refine understanding of the phenomenon'.

To view phenomena as the synthesised or elaborated essence of the subjects' experiencings is commonplace in the new phenomenology. Viewed in this way, phenomena are still on the level of subjective experience. Indeed, these researchers go to some pains to state that expressly. This has implications for the understanding of phenomenology. The basic and straightforward concept of phenomenon understands it as the object of experience — an understanding that has the propensity to introduce a note of objectivity into the discussion of phenomenology. If, however, the target of phenomenological research is purely the subjective experience of the respondents and not the phenomenon experienced, or if the phenomenon referred to is itself conceived in totally subjective terms, even identified with subjective experience as such, phenomenology is being understood and proposed as a project concerned exclusively with subjectivity.

The language used by these researchers encourages a thoroughly subjectivist interpretation of this kind. Even the word 'perception', which is capable of signifying the object of our perceiving, i.e. the 'object perceived', turns out in most cases to signify the act of perceiving. The researcher is interested in how this person perceives and what that way of perceiving implies for them and about them. The focus remains on the subject. The purpose of the research is to learn about the subjects of the research — about their perceiving, their feeling, their adoption of attitudes — rather than about what is perceived, the emotion felt, or the object towards which an attitude is taken.

In short, despite talk of 'phenomena' and despite the occurrence in some articles of what could be described as genuine, if fleeting, 'phenomenological moments', the phenomenology of these researchers remains overwhelmingly a study of subjective experience. Quite clearly, the task proposed here for phenomenology is that of identifying subjective experience, describing it and understanding it. In nursing research, what the phenomenological approach calls for, above all and before all, is a method of inquiry that will not prejudice the subjectivity of the experience under study. It demands a mode of data collection and data analysis that will present the participants' experience precisely from their particular perspective, i.e. in terms of the significance it has for them personally. What is sought is a first-person description that stays in the first person.

Given this task, the first enemy to be confronted is the researcher's own standpoint.

Bracketing

As the authors under consideration here make clear, researchers bring a great deal of intellectual 'baggage' to the tasks they undertake. Obtaining genuinely subjective data from the research participants and preserving its subjective character throughout the process of analysis may be the paramount concern, but researchers cannot deny that they all come armed with 'prior knowledge',[56] their own 'beliefs'[57] and 'judgements',[58] 'preconceived ideas and theories',[59] or 'personal and theoretic bias'.[60]

If we all have 'preconceptions and presuppositions',[61] how can we avoid imposing such presuppositions and preconceptions on the data?

The answer, according to several of the authors,[62] lies in 'bracketing' (a term introduced into phenomenology by Edmund Husserl). We need to bracket our presuppositions and preconceptions. Others among our authors[63] use alternative terms: they talk of 'suspending' our beliefs and assumptions, 'setting them aside', making ourselves 'as free as possible' from them, and so on. Lethbridge suggests that bracketing involves investigators' reflection on their past and current experiences so as to keep the meaning of those personal experiences separate from those revealed by the participants.[64]

In talking of this process, some expressly invoke Husserl[65] or refer to one or other of Husserl's commentators or fellow phenomenologists.[66]

What does bracketing achieve? The authors of these studies believe it achieves a great deal. The process makes it possible for researchers to focus on the respondents' experience.[67] While allowing informants to construct and give meaning to their own reality, it enables researchers to gain entry into the conceptual world of those informants[68] and discern it fully.[69] In this way, the data are accepted uncritically as given.[70] They are not tainted.[71]

According to Lethbridge,[72] and she refers to Omery[73] here, one of the practical implications of bracketing is that 'the question under study be examined with no operational definitions'. Nor, say Newman and Moch, should attention be paid to types or categories already identified in the literature.[74]

Among our authors are some who query whether one's presuppositions can be so definitely put aside or suspended. As the 'starting point for this phenomenologic study', Hauck is content simply to *identify* 'investigator assumptions' rather than rid herself of them.[75] Others seem to bow even more to the inevitable: Montbriand and Laing acknowledge that 'the researcher's frames of reference are imbedded in the interpretation',[76] while Zerwekh acknowledges that 'the author's frame of reference influences the process'.[77]

Such doubting Thomases aside, it is clear that, for most adherents of this kind of phenomenology, bracketing constitutes the starting point for research. In their terms, bracketing is a sincere endeavour not to allow one's beliefs and assumptions to shape the data collection process and a persistent effort not to impose one's own understandings and constructions on the data. Instead, the data must be allowed to emerge in their own form and 'speak for themselves'.

Phenomenological data collection

The emphasis on phenomenology varies from author to author. Some claim to be phenomenological from start to finish. Others invoke the phenomenological approach only when speaking of the way in which they glean their data or only when describing their data analysis method. Even within such specific areas the emphasis can vary significantly. This proves to be the case with data collection.

In gathering their data, what phenomenologically oriented nurse researchers are trying to ensure is that the subjective character of the data is left intact and untainted. It is only too easy for researchers to structure the data-gathering process in ways that virtually guarantee them the data they are after. Most investigators laying claim to a 'phenomenological approach' set out very deliberately to avoid this.

For one thing, they pay attention to the way in which they conduct their interviews. The authors in our collection talk about using 'un-structured',[78] 'semi-structured'[79] or 'open-ended'[80] interviews. This has to do with the questions that are put to the respondents. Where a 'structured' interview follows a standard questionnaire involving a set number of questions, these researchers have very few predetermined questions (Wood thinks that 'in true phenomenological research only one question is usually asked to elicit data')[81] and allow the interview to develop in spontaneous fashion. Watson describes this kind of interviewing:

The dialogue tends to be circular rather than linear; the descriptive questions employed flow from the course of the dialogue and not from a predetermined path. The interview is intended to yield a conversation, not a question/answer session.[82]

Not only is the interview open-ended in this sense but it tends to use open-ended questions.[83] Several of the researchers are chary about asking questions at all, adopting non-directive techniques[84] such as 'active listening',[85] 'frequent "um hums" ... Reflective silences and repetition of statements ... refocusing responses'.[86] Many point out that, beyond the opening question or two, further questions are asked only to gain clarification or encourage the respondent to keep talking.

The opening question or questions are designed to elicit descriptions of subjective experience. A manner of proceeding that appears very apt to a number of the authors is to ask the respondents to describe a situation.

- 'Please describe a situation in which you experienced postpartum depression.'[87]
- 'Describe a typical day in your home.'[88]
- 'Describe the most meaningful persons and events in your life.'[89]
- 'Can you tell me about a time when you felt stressed by what happened to you in hospital?'[90]
- 'Tell me about a situation in which you experienced a feeling of health.'[91]
- 'Tell about a time you will never forget because it reminds you of what it means to be a teacher or student in nursing today.'[92]

When asked to describe a situation in this way, the subjects may be invited specifically to share 'thoughts, perceptions, and feelings about the situation'.[93] This request to share 'thoughts', 'perceptions', 'views', 'insights', 'concerns' or 'feelings' is often put in its own right too, i.e. independently of the describe-a-situation gambit.[94] In either case, the informants may be asked to describe these ideas or sentiments until they 'have no more to say about the situation'[95] or have 'finished or exhausted their descriptions of the phenomenon'.[96] The researchers obviously consider thoughts, perceptions and feelings to be very much what phenomenology is about.

One way in which the authors go about asking their respondents to share their thoughts, perceptions and feelings about a situation is to ask them, 'What was it like?'[97] or 'What does it mean to you?'[98] These have come to be seen more or less as *the* phenomenological questions. (The 'to you', it may be suggested, is significant. Similarly, the question 'What was it like?' is understood here as 'What was it like *for you*?' rather than 'What was *it* like?' Rose, for example, asks her participants, 'What is inner strength like for you?')

Describing situations and events is a form of story telling and, for several of the authors,[99] the narrative mode stands forth as an ideal form for describing personal experiences.

> Story telling is emerging as a powerful qualitative strategy for understanding taken-for-granted practical knowledge ... The perspective of this study was phenomenologic, seeking to understand human experience through dialogue with ordinary people ... The nurse-researcher using this approach seeks to elucidate through dialogue turned into written text the clinical wisdom embedded in the everyday practice stories of nurses ... Applying common assumptions of naturalistic inquiry, this study explored the practice world through the rich narratives of expert public health nurses ... All nurses were asked to tell about one or more anecdotes ... They were urged to use the language of stories, not the usual abbreviated, case-reporting style.[100]

What these authors are attempting to develop are forms of data collection that both invite and facilitate authentic accounts of subjective experiences. The next task is to analyse these accounts without distorting them.

Phenomenological data analysis

Many of the articles detail a step-by-step process for analysing their data. Quite a number of the authors have adopted, and in most cases adapted, methods developed by Colaizzi,[101] Giorgi[102] and van Kaam.[103] Their interpretations, adaptations and fusions of such methods result in approaches along the following lines:

A Colaizzi-style method:

- reading the descriptions
- extracting 'significant statements'
- formulating meanings
- organising formulated meanings into clusters of themes
- exhaustively describing the investigated phenomenon
- validating the exhaustive description by each respondent.

A Giorgi-style method:

- initially listening to audiotapes and reading of transcripts to get a sense of the whole
- intuiting about, and reflecting on, each transcript
- identifying meaning units in each transcript
- regrouping and redescribing statements relevant to each meaning unit for each transcript

- intuiting about, and reflecting on, each meaning unit across all participants to uncover themes
- writing an 'exemplary narrative' to illustrate each invariant theme
- validating (by the participants and colleagues)
- synthesising statements.

A van Kaam-style method:

- listing descriptive expressions, their preliminary grouping into categories, and ranking categories by frequency of occurrence
- reducing descriptive expressions to more precise terms
- eliminating irrelevant expressions or elements
- formulating a hypothetical identification of the phenomenon
- applying the hypothetical description to randomly chosen cases of the sample, revising the hypothetical description in the light of this testing, and retesting on further samples
- finally identifying the description.

These approaches, as well as those which draw on different sources for their methods or devise their own, display a common concern to derive *themes* or *categories* from the data, which coalesce to form a *comprehensive description* of the total phenomenon.

In keeping with the emphasis on obtaining and maintaining truly subjective data, the themes should in no way be categories imposed upon the data. They are meant to arise from the data themselves. To enable this to happen, the researcher 'intuits' the data, as some of the authors put it.[104] By reflecting on the data, the researcher expects to uncover common themes that stem from the 'significant statements' or 'meaning units'.

The danger of imposing interpretations on the data is ever present. For this reason, some of the data-analysis systems used by the authors have inbuilt precautions. One such precaution is to have other people review the process. This may involve the formal use of a research team[105] or it may mean having 'another researcher with expertise in the field of phenomenology'[106] check out the categorisations and interpretations. Another precaution lies in returning, perhaps more than once, to the data[107] and to the participants[108] to check the validity of the interpretations.

Respecting the subjective

In this opening chapter the objective has been to discover the picture of phenomenology inherent in these thirty accounts of nursing research.

What has emerged is a single-minded effort to identify, describe and understand the subjective experience of respondents. Because the individual character of the data is always vulnerable owing to the ever-present danger of imposing extraneous meanings and constructions upon them, nursing phenomenologists deliberately prepare both themselves and their data-collection and data-analysis methods for the task. They prepare themselves by the process of bracketing — a self-conscious endeavour to hold their own preconceptions and presuppositions in abeyance. They prepare a data-collection process that does not guide subjects down predetermined paths but assists them to describe their individual experiences authentically and fully. They prepare a data-analysis process that attempts to preclude any imposition of interpretations from without but allows themes to emerge from the data as spontaneously as possible.

Looked at individually, not all of our authors set out to persist with this process all the way through, nor have all of them done what they planned to do with equal success. Nevertheless, taken together, they have proved a rich vein to mine.

The value of research done in this fashion needs no defending. Learning and understanding people's subjective experiences has an obvious and multi-faceted importance, as well as very practical applications, not least in a 'helping' profession such as nursing.

Accordingly, it is in no spirit of negative criticism that the question is raised: To what extent, if any, is this research phenomenological? As stated in the Introduction, Spiegelberg has referred to the 'common core' one needs to find in all phenomenologies in order to justify the use of the common label. Can we find it in this sort of phenomenology?

This is no idle question. Pickles has underscored the way in which his fellow geographers not only adopted phenomenology but radically adapted it to their own ends, a process issuing in the emergence of a 'geographical phenomenology' distinguishable from 'the precise and original meaning of phenomenology'.[109] In the same vein it is justifiable to speak of 'nursing phenomenology'. A certain understanding of phenomenology has come to the fore in nursing and now stands more or less as an orthodoxy for nurse researchers. What Pickles writes of geographical phenomenology holds for nursing phenomenology too: this is often the *only* phenomenology to which subsequent writers turn.

The parallel with geography is not total. Unlike what Pickles claims for geographers, it is not the case that nurse researchers have developed their own phenomenology. Rather, they have avidly embraced a form of phenomenology which developed around them and which appears to serve their purposes well. Nevertheless, the question remains: if nursing phenomenology, like the form of phenomenology from which it derives, is a substantial adaptation of mainstream phenomenology, does the one now coincide at all with the other? The question has its importance. After all, if these are indeed distinct methodologies, it is conceivable that a more traditional form of phenomenology could also serve the purposes of nursing research. Perhaps it would do so in equally useful ways. It might even do so in ways that are more useful. Let us see whether this is so. We have considered nursing phenomenology. We need now to look to mainstream phenomenology and identify what makes it what it is.

NOTES

1 Anderson (1991b), p. 1.
2 The thirty articles are listed in boxes on pp. 10–11.
3 The selection was made by the CINAHL CD-ROM disk! A listing of articles with 'phenomenology' in the descriptors was requested. The thirty articles used here are the first thirty occurring on the list which were available and expressly laid claim to being phenomenological in approach.
4 See Diekelmann (1992), Dobbie (1991), Rather (1992), Watson (1991), Zerwekh (1992).
5 All but Eyres et al. (1992), Mason (1992), McHaffie (1991), Monahan (1992), and Montbriand and Laing (1991) expressly relate phenomenology to 'experience'.
6 See Beck (1991a, 1991b, 1992), Bennett (1991), Breault and Polifroni (1992), Diekelmann (1992), Elfert et al. (1991), Henderson and Brouse (1991), Lethbridge (1991), Marr (1991), Rather (1992), Rose (1990), Whetstone and Reid (1991), Wolf (1991), Wondolowski and Davis (1991), Zerwekh (1992).
7 See Beck (1991a, 1991b), Elfert et al. (1991), Lethbridge (1991), Rather (1992), Rose (1990), Wondolowski and Davis (1991).
8 See Beck (1992), Bennett (1991), Diekelmann (1992), Elfert et al. (1991), Rather (1992), Rose (1990), Zerwekh (1992).
9 See Beck (1991a, 1991b), Bowman (1991), Dobbie (1991), Lethbridge (1991), Rose (1990), Wondolowski and Davis (1991).
10 See Anderson (1991a), Zerwekh (1992).
11 See Bennett (1991), Breault and Polifroni (1992), Elfert et al. (1991), Eyres et al. (1992), Hauck (1991), Keefe and Froese-Fretz (1991), Lethbridge (1991), Marr (1991), Mason (1992), Montbriand and Laing (1991), Rather (1992), Wolf (1991).
12 See Anderson (1991a), Dobbie (1991), Elfert et al. (1991), Lethbridge (1991), Martin (1991), Mason (1992), Wolf (1991), Wondolowski and Davis (1991), Zerwekh (1992).
13 See Bowman (1991), Marr (1991), Martin (1991), Rose (1990).
14 Watson (1991), p. 11.
15 Zerwekh (1992), p. 16.
16 Wolf (1991), p. 75.
17 Rather (1992), p. 48.
18 Wolf (1991), p. 75.
19 Breault and Polifroni (1992, p. 23) chose the phenomenological methodology so as 'to identify and describe the experience of caring', while Watson (1991, p. 10) aimed to identify experiences to be eliminated, modified or promoted in practice.
20 Experience is to be studied (Beck, Bennett, Watson), researched (Diekelmann), explored (Beck, Keefe and Froese-Fretz, Marr), examined (Marr, Wolf), investigated (Wolf).
21 See Anderson (1991a), p. 710.

22 Phenomenology seeks to understand the nature of experiences (Beck, Wolf), their meaning (Beck, Bennett, Diekelmann, Dobbie, Elfert et al., Rose, Wolf, Wondolowski and Davis), their structure (Bennett, Rose) or essential structure (Beck, Wolf).

23 Dobbie (1991), p. 825.

24 Rather (1992), p. 48.

25 See Bennett (1991), p. 437.

26 Phenomenology's aim is to describe experience (Beck, Bennett, Elfert et al., Lethbridge, Marr, Martin, Wondolowski and Davis, Wood) — at least a 'specific domain of experience (Watson 1991, p. 11) — with its essential structure (Beck) and the participants' 'thoughts and feelings ... within the context of their own subjective experience' (Martin 1991, p. 494).

27 Wolf (1991), p. 74.

28 Breault and Polifroni (1992), p. 21.

29 *Ibid.*, p. 22.

30 The experience on which the research focuses is:
- a feeling of uselessness (Anderson)
- the psychological state of depression (Beck 1992)
- a feeling of being cared for (Beck 1991a)
- a feeling of health (Beck 1991b)
- 'feelings and attitudes' (Breault and Polifroni 1992, pp. 21, 22)
- 'intense emotions', 'expectations', reactions 'when reality began to intrude', feelings of comfort and being in charge (Henderson and Brouse 1991, pp. 295–296)
- the feeling of health by the oldest old, entailing vitality, fulfilment and 'rhapsodic reverie' (Wondolowski and Davis)

31 Experience is presented as:
- the locus in which 'the frequently taken for granted shared practices and common meanings [are] embedded' (Diekelmann 1992, p. 73)
- 'an evolving consciousness of self and children, and an evolving consciousness of God' (Dobbie 1991, p. 827)
- 'parents' views of their child' (Elfert et al. 1991, p. 116).

32 The experience which the research seeks to study is:
- 'feelings, thoughts and perceptions' (Rose 1990, p. 60)
- perceptions ['brain-dead patient transformed into organ donor'], attitudes [a sense of 'dual responsibility to donor and recipient families'] and feelings [nurses 'are saddened by the donor's death' and there are 'emotional reactions to organ procurement surgery and the events surrounding the surgery'] (Wolf 1991, pp. 78–86)
- 'thoughts, perceptions and feelings about perceived barriers to hypertensive health promotion' (Whetstone and Reid 1991, p. 1344).

33 Events — what happens to people — constitutes 'experience' for
- Hauck (the toileting process)
- Watson (hospitalisation due to psychiatric illness).

34 Experience means:
- the witnessing of marital violence and the effect it has on adolescent girls (Bennett)
- changes in people's total situation, together with their reactions to the changes (Bowman)
- the crisis situation caused by colic in an infant, including the effect on the mother (Keefe and Froese-Fretz)
- the use of contraception throughout women's fertile years and how the women perceived this and felt about it (Lethbridge)

- the development of Parkinson's disease and what this meant to the participants, especially their feelings about it (Marr)
- the development of adult polycystic kidney disease, together with the participants' 'thoughts and feelings about APKD within the context of their own subjective experience' (Martin 1991, p. 494).
- most meaningful events and persons, together with feelings and felt needs (Newman and Moch)

35 Rather speaks of schooling experiences, Wood of the experience of being a caregiver, and Zerwekh of nurses' everyday practice.
36 See Anderson (1991a), Beck (1991a, 1991b, 1992), Bennett (1991), Bowman (1991), Dobbie (1991), Elfert et al. (1991), Henderson and Brouse (1991), Marr (1991), Rather (1992), Wolf (1991).
37 Parse in Bowman (1991), p. 382.
38 Beck (1992), p. 167.
39 See Anderson (1991a), Beck (1991a, 1991b, 1992), Dobbie (1991), Rather (1992).
40 See Beck (1991b).
41 Bennett (1991), p. 432.
42 Elfert et al. (1991), p. 115.
43 Dobbie (1991), p. 826.
44 See Bowman (1991), p. 382.
45 Bennett (1991), p. 432.
46 Bowman (1991), p. 382
47 Marr (1991), p. 325.
48 Wolf (1991), p. 74.
49 Beck (1991a), p. 19.
50 Henderson and Brouse (1991), p. 294.
51 Beck (1991b), p. 373.
52 Marr (1991), p. 325.
53 Rose (1990), p. 60.
54 Wolf (1991), p. 74.
55 Omery (1983), p. 61.
56 Rose (1990), p. 59.
57 Beck (1991a), p. 19.
58 Dobbie (1991), p. 826.
59 Lethbridge (1991), p. 276.
60 Rose (1990), p. 59.
61 Beck (1992), p. 167.
62 See Beck (1991a, 1992), Keefe and Froese-Fretz (1991), Lethbridge (1991), Rose (1990).
63 See Bowman (1991), Breault and Polifroni (1992), Dobbie (1991), Hauck (1991), Montbriand and Laing (1991), Newman and Moch (1991), Wolf (1991), Zerwekh (1992).
64 See Lethbridge (1991), p. 277.
65 See Montbriand and Laing (1991), Rose (1990).
66 Beck (1992) refers the notion to Spiegelberg; Zerwekh (1992) refers to Heidegger.
67 See Dobbie (1991), p. 826.
68 See Montbriand and Laing (1991), p. 327.
69 See Rose (1990), p. 59.
70 See Lethbridge (1991), p. 276.
71 See Rose (1990), p. 59.
72 Lethbridge (1991), p. 276.

73 See Omery (1983), p. 51.
74 See Newman and Moch (1991), p. 162.
75 Hauck (1991), p. 81.
76 Montbriand and Laing (1991), p. 327.
77 Zerwekh (1992), p. 16.
78 See Bennett (1991), Elfert et al. (1991), Keefe and Froese-Fretz (1991), Marr (1991), Rose (1990), Watson (1991).
79 See Hauck (1991), Henderson and Brouse (1991), Lethbridge (1991), Mason (1992), Wolf(1991), Wood (1991).
80 See Hauck (1991), Keefe and Froese-Fretz (1991), Marr (1991), Martin (1991), Mason (1992), Whetstone and Reid (1991).
81 Wood (1991), p. 196.
82 Watson (1991), p. 11.
83 See Hauck (1991), Marr (1991), Martin (1991), Whetstone and Reid (1991).
84 See Bennett (1991), Bowman (1991), Diekelmann (1992), Dobbie (1991), Hauck (1991), Martin (1991), Newman and Moch (1991), Rather (1992), Rose (1990), Watson (1991), Whetstone and Reid (1991).
85 Hauck (1991), p. 82.
86 Dobbie (1991), p. 826.
87 See Beck (1992), p. 167.
88 See Bennett (1991), p. 433.
89 See Newman and Moch (1991), p. 162.
90 See Watson (1991), p. 11.
91 See Wondolowski and Davis (1991), p. 114.
92 See Diekelmann (1992), p. 73.
93 See Beck (1991a. 1991b, 1992), Wondolowski and Davis (1991).
94 See Beck (1991a. 1991b, 1992), Eyres et al. (1992), Keefe and Froese-Fretz (1991), Martin (1991), Rose (1990), Whetstone and Reid (1991), Wolf (1991), Wondolowski and Davis (1991).
95 Beck (1991a), p. 19; (1991b), p. 372; (1992), p. 167.
96 Rose (1990), p. 60.
97 See Lethbridge (1991), Marr (1991), Rather (1992), Rose (1990), Whetstone and Reid (1991), Wood (1991).
98 See Diekelmann (1992), Newman and Moch (1991), Wood (1991).
99 See Anderson (1991a), Diekelmann (1992), Dobbie (1991), Zerwekh (1992).
100 Zerwekh (1992), p. 16
101 See Beck (1991a, 1992), Rose (1990), Wolf (1991), citing Colaizzi (1978).
102 See Bennett (1991), Bowman (1991), Dobbie (1991), Henderson and Brouse (1991), citing Giorgi (1970, 1971, 1975a, 1975b, 1985).
103 See Beck (1991b), Wondolowski and Davis (1991), citing Van Kaam (1966).
104 See Dobbie (1991), Lethbridge (1991), Rose (1990), Wondolowski and Davis (1991).
105 See Diekelmann (1992), Elfert et al (1991), Martin (1991), Rather (1992).
106 Bowman (1991), p. 382. See Beck (1991b, 1992), Dobbie (1991), Eyres et al. (1992), Montbriand and Laing (1991), Wondolowski and Davis (1991), Zerwekh (1992).
107 See Beck (1991a, 1991b), Diekelmann (1992), Dobbie (1991), Rather (1992), Rose (1990), Wolf (1991).
108 See Beck (1991a, 1992), Diekelmann (1992), Dobbie (1991), Montbriand and Laing (1991), Newman and Moch (1991), Rather (1992), Rose (1990), Wolf (1991).
109 Pickles (1985), p. 5.

2

'Back to the things themselves'

The word 'phenomenology' has a long and tortuous history. Today, however, at least when used to denote a philosophy or approach, it tends to be taken for 'the project of Edmund Husserl and its subsequent development'.[1] While this subsequent development led phenomenology far from the original project, it constitutes an identifiable approach to knowledge and reality and is not infrequently referred to as a 'movement'.

What Husserl (1859–1938), phenomenology's acknowledged founder, sought to establish was a secure basis for human knowledge. He spoke of his need for clarity, referring to 'torments' he had gone through 'from lack of clarity and from doubt'.[2] Accordingly, he looked for principles on which all science, in the broadest sense, could be built. It was a quest that led him, as a mathematician first of all, to be concerned with the logical foundations of his discipline and then to abandon mathematics for philosophy. The philosophy he sought was to be above all 'a science of Beginnings, a "first" philosophy', such that 'all philosophical disciplines, the very foundations of all science whatsoever, spring from its matrix'.[3] It was a quest that consumed his life to the end.

What this means is that Husserl was interested in laying foundations rather than building an edifice. He never developed a systematic philosophy. Instead of creating a system to stand alongside other systems, he yearned to establish such a clear and secure basis for human knowledge that the very existence of different 'systems' would be unthinkable. It was in this vein that he wrote in 1933 to an American correspondent, E Parl Welch:

> May I ask you not to call my philosophy a 'system'. For it is precisely its objective to make all 'systems' impossible once and for all. It wants to be rigorous science ...[4]

It means, secondly, that Husserl saw himself as standing alone. Because he was concerned with 'first philosophy' (the title of one of his lecture series and of a posthumous publication based on that series), he could not borrow concepts, let alone principles, from his philosophical predecessors. In this respect he identified with Descartes and placed these words on Descartes' lips:

> I, the solitary individual philosophizer, owe much to others; but what they accept as true, what they offer me as allegedly established by their insight, is for me at first only something they claim. If I am to accept it, I must justify it by a perfect insight on my own part. Therein consists my autonomy — mine and that of every genuine scientist.[5]

It means, furthermore, that for Husserl the task could never end. Throughout his life, he continued to explore the foundations ever more profoundly. He was never satisfied. Such was his passion for clarity that his many published works turn out to be little else than a long series of 'Introductions' to his phenomenology. For him, philosophy is a perpetual beginning — a viewpoint that some of the later representatives of the phenomenological movement would certainly share. Merleau-Ponty (who once described himself as a 'perpetual beginner') and Ricoeur are examples of this. Although, as phenomenologists, they were to travel in a significantly different direction from Husserl, they agree that the path has no end.[6]

In the face of a project like that, the starting point assumes critical importance.

Search for reality

Where did Husserl believe the foundations or principles of knowledge are to be found? Not, to be sure, in speculative principles drawn from the philosophies of the past. Certainly not within the framework of established metaphysics. Not, in fact, in anything at all that is taken for granted. Instead, for Husserl, the first step was to take a fresh look at the reality he wanted to understand and explain. In this spirit he launched his program under the battle cry of *Zu den Sachen selbst*, 'Back to the things themselves'.[7] To ground knowledge about reality, he looked to reality itself.

This hardly sounds like a call to subjectivism. Although the reality Husserl looked to was reality *as it presents itself to human consciousness*, he refused to divorce reality from consciousness—a refusal that was to become the hallmark of phenomenologists of whatever stripe. Consciousness held a lifelong fascination for Husserl. 'The wonder of all wonders,' he was to say, 'is the pure Ego and pure consciousness.'[8] While his fascination with consciousness led him more and more into a transcendental idealism, he never lost sight of the reality he was seeking through consciousness. *Zu den Sachen selbst* may have come to be more aptly expressed as *Wende zum Gegenstand* ('Turn to the object'), but either way the emphasis on gaining knowledge of reality remained firm. Husserl may, in the end, have rejected most forms of realism, but reality remained his goal. Spiegelberg puts it this way:

> ... Husserl's enterprise may well be characterized as the triumph of objectivity over subjectivity, or better as the establishment of objectivity in the very heart of subjectivity.[9]

In 1913, when Husserl wrote an introduction to the second edition of his *Logical Investigations*, he reflected on what he had attempted to do in the second volume of that work. His efforts there, he said, had to do with 'things' (as he would later prefer to put it, his search was for the 'object'). If he turned to the subject, to consciousness, it was because it was there he expected to encounter the object he was after.

> For if these Investigations are to prove helpful to those interested in phenomenology, this will be because they do not offer us a mere programme (certainly not one of the high-flying sort which so encumber philosophy) but that they are attempts at genuinely executed fund–amental work on the immediately envisaged and seized things themselves. Even where they proceed critically, they do not lose themselves in discussions of standpoint, but rather leave the last word to the things themselves and to one's work upon such things.[10]

Martin Heidegger (1889–1976), Husserl's colleague and successor at the University of Freiburg, looked to the 'things themselves' too. Since Heidegger did not follow his phenomenological mentor down the path of transcendental idealism but is generally accredited with giving phen-omenology its earliest existentialist setting,[11] this is hardly surprising.

> Thus the term 'phenomenology' expresses a maxim which can be formulated as 'To the things themselves!'. It is opposed to all free-floating constructions and accidental findings; it is opposed to taking over any conceptions which only seem to have been demonstrated; it is opposed to those pseudo-questions which parade themselves as 'problems', often for generations at a time.[12]

The subjective quality of all knowledge goes without saying. That notwithstanding, the task of philosophical analysis, for Husserlian phenomenologists and existential phenomenologists alike, is to uncover essential structures of reality.[13] We must let the 'things themselves' be our guide, as Kockelmans points out:

> Phenomenology indicates primarily a principle of method, which can best be formulated in Husserl's phrase: 'Back to the things themselves.' This expression ... indicates that in philosophy one should renounce all principles and ideas that are insufficiently explained or incorrectly founded, all arbitrary ways of thinking and all prejudices, and be guided only by the things themselves.[14]

31

Phenomenological method

This return to the 'things themselves' — this search for reality — is difficult to square with the overriding subjectivism of the new phenomenology as exemplified, say, in nursing research. In nursing phenomenology, the quest is for people's subjective perceptions, thoughts and feelings rather than for what is objective, i.e. the phenomena, revealed in and through them.

This contrast is pointed up when one compares the actions taken in nursing phenomenology, described in the last chapter, with the phenomenological method outlined by Spiegelberg.[15] Spiegelberg lists for us seven elements of phenomenological method. Spiegelberg originally called these 'steps', which led some of his readers to equate the outline with stepwise data-analysis methods like those considered in Chapter 1.[16] What Spiegelberg is doing, however, is listing actions that various phenomenologists have taken. It is, he tells us, 'an attempt to formulate the core and the periphery of the varieties of phenomenology'. He regards the first three actions as essential: all aligned with the phenomenological movement accept these, at least implicitly. A smaller number of phenomenologists have practised some or all of the other elements.

The seven elements listed by Spiegelberg are these:

1 Investigating particular phenomena
This involves intuition, analysis and description of phenomena. By investigating phenomena Spiegelberg means going 'to the things themselves', i.e. to the objects of immediate experience. He makes it clear that phenomena do not include 'crystallized beliefs and theories handed down by a tradition which only too often perpetuates preconceptions and prejudgments'. These inherited understandings adulterate the phenomena and are to be excluded from consideration. What Spiegelberg is outlining is a process of 'identification and deliberate elimination of theoretical constructs and symbolisms in favor of the return to the unadulterated phenomena'. Phenomenology, he tells us, is an 'unusually obstinate attempt to look at the phenomena and to remain faithful to them before even thinking about them'.

2 Investigating general essences
The intuiting of particular phenomena provides the general essences. As the particular phenomena are considered, there emerges an affinity, a structural similarity, a pervading essence. This permeates the particular phenomena and is expressed through them. (This process is known as eidetic description. To designate a universal essence, Husserl made use of the Greek word *eidos*, which Plato had employed as an alternative for 'idea' or 'form'. From this comes the adjective 'eidetic'.)

3 Apprehending essential relationships
The relationships referred to exist within an essence or between essences.

4 Watching modes of appearing

Phenomenology, Spiegelberg suggests, involves the systematic exploration of phenomena not only in the sense of what appears but also of the way in which things appear.

5 Exploring the constitution of phenomena in consciousness

This means determining the way in which a phenomenon establishes itself and takes shape in our consciousness.

6 Suspending belief in existence

Suspending belief in the existence of the phenomena, according to Spiegelberg, enables the phenomenologist to concentrate on the non-existential, i.e. essential content, the 'what' of the phenomena.

7 Interpreting concealed meanings

This is included by Spiegelberg, somewhat reluctantly, in view of the hermeneutical approaches adopted by philosophers such as Heidegger, Merleau-Ponty, Sartre and Ricoeur. In this process. 'the interpreter has to go beyond what is directly given. In attempting this, he has to use the given as a clue for meanings which are not given, or at least not explicitly given'.

The actions proposed here by Spiegelberg relate to phenomena, i.e. the objects of our experience, and not to subjective reactions. He makes it abundantly clear that phenomenology has no interest in the '"merely subjective" observations which characterize the reports of uncritical and untrained observers chosen at random'.[17] (These are, of course, the very observations which the new phenomenologists are concerned to gather as the data of their research.) It is true that the phenomenologist never loses sight of the subject and the subject's consciousness. It is true that phenomenological analysis involves both the act of the subject (the *noetic* dimension) and the content or object of the act (the *noematic* dimension). Nevertheless, the ultimate goal of phenomenology is clearly the elucidation of phenomena. The phenomenon, Spiegelberg insists, 'is to be studied for its own sake, regardless of the specific case'.[18]

Further confirmation can be found in the writings of the Duquesne University phenomenologist, Adrian van Kaam. As we have seen, his method is followed by some of the nursing researchers under consideration in Chapter 1. However, van Kaam cannot be invoked on the side of subjectivism. In his work as a psychologist, he sees several forms of subjectivism into which he might fall.

> I call such approaches subjectivistic because they arise not from my observations of objective reality but from an *a priori* concept which I, the subject, hold about reality.
>
> The main source of my subjectivism is my refusal to open myself first to the phenomena as they are given to me ...[19]

It is this openness to 'the phenomena as they are given' that informs van Kaam's method. It is not about describing subjective thoughts, attitudes or feelings on the part of particular subjects for their own sake. It is about describing phenomena. This is shown in very direct fashion when van Kaam talks of selecting subjects for his research, which is a study of the phenomenon of 'being understood'. There are subjects, obviously, for whom being understood is a problem. It will be in the interests of those subjects, and others in similar situations, if the researcher can study them and gain insight into how they perceive their problem with being understood and the feelings they have about it. This is the kind of research that nursing phenomenologists tend to embark upon. Not so van Kaam. He does not choose subjects of that kind. Instead, he selects 'the best group of subjects available in our culture for the prescientific explication of the human experience of really feeling understood'. The phenomenon on which he is focusing is a human feeling, i.e. the sense of 'being understood'. For his study he wants people who are able to express not only 'their inner feelings and emotions without shame and inhibition' but also 'the organic experiences that accompany these feelings'. As we shall see in Chapter 3, the phenomena of phenomenology are not just *any* experiences or, to put it more accurately, not just any level of experiences. That is what van Kaam's 'prescientific explication' and 'organic experiences' refer to. It is very clear that his immediate interest does not lie in determining subjective experiences in terms of particular subjects or for the sake of particular subjects. He wants to delineate a phenomenon. He chooses subjects for the sake of phenomena, not phenomena for the sake of subjects.[20] He is in hot pursuit of what he has termed 'objective reality'.[21]

This is true also of other methodologists invoked by the nursing researchers examined in Chapter 1, e.g. Giorgi and Colaizzi. They too look for a description of phenomena. Describing the lifeworld as 'the world as we live it prior to any reflection upon it as such', Giorgi explains that 'the significance of the lifeworld for the approach to psychology is that psychology must account for its phenomena in terms of how they appear, or how they are experienced'.[22]

Max van Manen, who is cited by Diekelmann and Rose, is very explicit. He uses the phenomenological study of parenting as an example:

> From a phenomenological point of view we are not primarily interested in the subjective experiences of our so-called subjects or informants, for the sake of being able to report on how something is seen from their particular point of view, perspective or vantage point. Of course, we may want to know what mothering or fathering is like from the viewpoint of the single parent, or the bereaved parent, or from the perspective of working-class parents or more well-to-do parents who employ nannies or babysitters, and so forth. However, the deeper goal,

which is always the thrust of phenomenological research, remains oriented to asking the question of what is the nature of this phenomenon (parenting) as an essentially human experience ... No matter how any particular parent (or group of parents) relates to a child, we always want to know: How is this parenting? Is this what it is like to parent? Is this what it means to be a mother or father?[23]

It is this focus on the phenomenon — this asking of what van Manen calls 'the essential phenomenological question' — that, in his view, distinguishes phenomenology from 'other so-called qualitative research approaches (such as ethnography, ethnomethodology, symbolic interactionism, conceptual analysis, biography, etc.)'. We need, he insists, to recognise the force of that question.

Clark Moustakas stands in this same tradition. He draws on phenomenology to articulate the 'heuristic inquiry' model which lies behind his well-known study of loneliness.[24] While Moustakas is interested in 'seeing what an experience *is* for another person, ... seeing attitudes, beliefs and feelings of the person as they exist for him at the moment he is experiencing them, perceiving them whole, as unity', his purpose is clear:

> I set out to know the meaning of loneliness, not by defining and categorizing, but by experiencing it directly and through the lives of others, as simple reality of life ... I set out to discover the meaning of loneliness in its simplest terms ... I was searching for, studying, and inquiring into the nature and impact of loneliness. I was totally involved and immersed in this search for a pattern and meaning which would reveal the various dimensions of loneliness in modern life ... I steeped myself in a world of loneliness, letting my life take root and unfold in it, letting its dimensions and meanings and forms evolve its own timetable and dynamics ... When a pattern began to emerge with reference to the nature and function of loneliness in individual experience and in modern living, the formal study came to an end. At this point the framework and detail, the clarification of loneliness, had been formed; it was possible to differentiate and refine its meaning, to expand and illustrate its nature and relevance in human experience.[25]

The 'meaning of loneliness', the 'nature and impact of loneliness', 'a pattern and meaning which would reveal the various dimensions of loneliness', 'its dimensions and meanings and forms', the 'nature and function of loneliness', 'its nature and relevance' — it is a constant refrain and it leaves no doubt about this researcher's intent. What Moustakas is seeking to elucidate is loneliness and not just lonely people.

Moustakas was led to study loneliness through personal experience. This related to his daughter's health and, because it brought him into contact with children in hospital, he began to observe their loneliness too. He did not rest content with describing how he or these children experienced loneliness. His study became phenomenological as he moved from an understanding of their individual experience of loneliness to an insight into what makes loneliness loneliness. As he puts it, 'what started as a hospital study of loneliness became an extended research into the phenomenon of loneliness'.[26] What he gained was 'an intuitive grasping of the patterns of loneliness, of related aspects and associations, until an integrated vision and awareness emerged'.[27]

With Moustakas, then, as with the other authors cited, phenomenology remains, above all else, a search for reality. It is not just a study of subjects. What it studies in the subjects is the *object* of their experience, so that there is an objectivity about phenomenological research. Thévenaz even calls phenomenology an 'extreme objectivism'. It may be 'an adventure of consciousness' but, he insists, 'this does not detract in any way from the extreme objectivism of this philosophy, an objectivism that remains a constant throughout the course of this long and multiple effort of going back "to the things themselves"'.[28]

Bochenski writes in the same vein. In phenomenology, he says, it 'is imperative to get at *the things themselves*'. This is 'the first and fundamental rule in the phenomenological method'.[29]

> The phenomenological method is neither deductive nor empirical, but consists in *pointing (Aufweis)* to what is given and *elucidating* it; it neither explains by means of laws nor deduces from any principles, instead it fixes its gaze directly upon whatever is presented to consciousness, that is, its object. Consequently its whole direction is toward the objective, and although the activity of a subject can itself become an object of investigation in its own right, it is neither this activity nor the subjective concept which immediately interests the phenomenologist but rather what is known, doubted, loved, hated, and so forth.[30]

Behind this lies the concept of intentionality.

Intentionality

Intentionality is a notion Husserl gleaned from his teacher, Franz Brentano (1838–1917), with whom he studied at the University of Vienna. Brentano was an outstanding philosopher and psychologist, a charismatic figure whose influence was widespread and enduring. During 1884–86 Husserl spent four semesters at Vienna, attending all of Brentano's lecture courses and taking part in his seminars. At the end of the fourth semester Brentano invited Husserl to spend three months of the summer vacation with him.

In 1888–89 Brentano used the word 'phenomenology' as an alternative title for a course he presented on 'Descriptive psychology'. Perhaps it was from this that Husserl borrowed the word which he was to fill with such rich meaning. What he received from Brentano, however, was much more than a word.

For a start, it was under Brentano's influence that Husserl moved definitively from mathematics to philosophy. In the process Brentano succeeded in inspiring Husserl with his own kind of passion for rigorous science. While Brentano saw himself as an empiricist ('Experience alone is my teacher') and his best known work is *Psychology from an Empirical Standpoint,* he felt that 'this is entirely compatible with a certain ideal point of view'.[31] Brentano was writing about psychology rather than philosophy, but one may still detect a foreshadowing of Husserl's phenomenology in this combination of experience and an ideal point of view. Moreover, in developing this phenomenology, Husserl came to share Brentano's intense interest in the relationship between consciousness and time. His lectures on 'Phenomenology of inner time consciousness', presented between 1905 and 1910, form a key component of the Husserlian corpus.

While Husserl owed to Brentano many elements in his development as a philosopher, there is no doubt at all that the most important contribution Brentano made to Husserl's philosophy was the concept of intentionality. In the letter to E Parl Welch referred to earlier, Husserl freely acknowledged Brentano's decisive influence and referred at once to this concept:

> My entire development is determined by the stimulation of Franz Brentano (my academic teacher) — by his psychology, which included intentionality as a fundamental character of the psychic.[32]

Intentionality was not a concept that Brentano had discovered within the prevailing German philosophy of his day. Brentano was a former Catholic priest. He drew the concept of intentionality from the Scholastic philosophy he was introduced to as he prepared for the priesthood. Scholasticism is the philosophy, basically Aristotelian, which was adopted and shaped by the medieval scholars such as Thomas Aquinas and developed, or debased, by their successors down the centuries. As Brentano wrestled with the problem of making a cogent distinction between physical and psychic phenomena, he saw intentionality as the answer.

> Every mental phenomenon is characterized by what the Scholastics of the Middle Ages called the intentional (or mental) in-existence[33] of an object, and what we might call, although not wholly unambiguously, reference to a content, direction toward an object (which is not to be understood here as meaning a thing), or immanent objectivity. Every mental phenomenon includes something as object within itself, although they do not all do so in the same way. In presentation something is presented, in judgment something is affirmed or denied, in love loved, in hate hated, in desire desired and so on.
>
> This intentional in-existence is characteristic exclusively of mental phenomena. No physical phenomenon exhibits anything like it. We can therefore define mental phenomena by saying that they are those phenomena which contain an object intentionally within themselves.[34]

37

The terms 'intentionality' and 'intentional' are difficult for us to grapple with because of their associations. It is not easy for us to lay aside the everyday meaning we attribute to them. As one author has put it, 'our words get in our eyes'.[35] The notion of 'purpose', 'what we deliberately plan to do', floods in upon us. That notion has nothing to do with intentionality as it is understood here. 'In-tending' in our present context is not about proposing or planning but about *reaching into* (just as '*extending*' is about *reaching out from*).

Intentionality evokes for us, therefore, the idea of the human mind reaching out and into the objects of which it is conscious. This is what Brentano is talking about when he speaks of 'reference to a content, direction toward an object' by which psychic phenomena are to be characterised. When he describes them as 'intentional', he means that they bear an essential relationship to an object. Intentionality means referentiality, relatedness, directedness.

The Scholastics had another way of expressing this. They said that the object of knowledge comes to dwell within the knower. *Cognitum est in cognoscente*: 'What is known is in the knower'. Not such a difficult concept, surely: in common parlance we often speak of things 'entering' our consciousness. Brentano is referring to this understanding of the knowledge process when he says that psychic phenomena have an 'intentional in-existence' or an 'immanent objectivity'. Each psychic phenomenon, he tells us, 'includes something as object within itself'.

The Scholastic philosophers, Brentano might also have mentioned, had yet another way of depicting the union of subject with object, this wedding of the knower to what is known. They claimed that to know something is, in a fashion, to *become* that something, i.e. to become something other than oneself and so transcend one's own self.[36]

In these various ways the Scholastics were positing a very intimate relationship between the subject and the object of the subject's consciousness. At the same time, they were attributing to consciousness an active role: the mind reaches out to the object and into the object and draws it into itself, at once shaping the object and being shaped by it. Such an intimate and dynamic role was not paralleled in the epistemologies prevailing in the late nineteenth century. In empiricist thought, such as that of Locke, consciousness is presented as empty and passive. In Kantian thought, the mind is seen as more active, it is true, but in a formal sense only, imposing the Kantian categories and in the process creating a barrier between consciousness and reality. As Kant would have it, we may know the appearances (*phenomena*) but we can never know the things in themselves (*noumena*). In contrast to these understandings, the Scholastic explanation offers human consciousness a genuine grasp on reality and it was clearly this that appealed to Brentano.[37]

In drawing on Scholasticism, Brentano did not refer to knowing as 'becoming something other than oneself'. And, in the end, he discarded the notion of 'in-existence'. He may well have come to regard that as too closely allied to other aspects of Scholastic epistemology which he would have no truck with. However, the idea that all psychic phenomena — and therefore consciousness itself — have 'reference to a content', a 'direction toward an object', is one that remained central to his thought.

It was this idea which Husserl had already taken from Brentano and which he came to regard as the pivotal insight of his philosophy. He dealt with intentionality for the first time in the second volume of his *Logical Investigations*. Gurwitsch writes that Husserl

> ... agrees with Brentano in acknowledging the existence of a highly
> important class of mental facts — for which Husserl reserves the title
> of acts — which have the peculiarity of presenting the subject with an
> object. Experiencing an act, the subject is aware of the object, so that
> the act may be characterized, as Husserl does, as a consciousness of an
> object whether real or ideal, whether existent or imaginary.[38]

Heidegger, too, was keenly aware of intentionality — and of its Scholastic origin, for Heidegger, like Brentano, had been well schooled in Scholasticism. Heidegger was briefly a Jesuit novice and then for some years a student for the priesthood in the Archdiocese of Freiburg. In 1915, when seeking admission to the University of Freiburg as a *Privatdozent*, the thesis he submitted dealt with the doctrine of the thirteenth-century Scholastic philosopher and theologian, Duns Scotus. In this work Heidegger recognises the need for Husserl-style emphasis on the noetic acts of consciousness to counterbalance what he saw as Scholasticism's overly objectivist epistemology. At the same time, he commends the Scholastic method for the scope it offers for phenomenological intuiting and the way in which it lends itself to the study of intentionality.

What is intentionality, then? It is the idea that, as Brentano pointed out, every thought is thought *of something*, every desire is a desire *of something*, and every judgment is an acceptance or rejection *of something*. Consciousness is always and essentially related to objects. In short, there is an indissoluble union between subject and object. Pickles underlines the centrality of this notion in phenomenological thought:

> There is one element common to all true phenomenologies since
> Husserl and that is their rejection of the traditional metaphysical
> assumption of the separation of subject and object as the description
> of the fundamental state of affairs ... This we can call the Cartesian or
> Newtonian world-view, and presupposes what Heidegger has called a
> pro-posing, positing form of thinking and interpreting the world, 'which
> *secures* beings as objects *over against itself and for itself* (Welte, 1982,
> 92).[39]

This is not to suggest that subject and object are the same. We must distinguish between them. We should not collapse the object into the subject, as some forms of idealism do, nor the subject into the object as some forms of realism do. But, distinct as they are, they are not thereby separate. Subject and object are bound up inextricably with one another, so that it makes sense to search in human consciousness for what Husserl terms 'objectivities'.

> ... every kind of theoretical, valuational, practical consciousness can be made in the same manner a theme for inquiry; and all the Objectivities constituted in it can be investigated.[40]

In more existentialist hands, the concept of intentionality ceases to be expressed in purely epistemological terms. It becomes ontological, if not anthropological. Not only is consciousness intentional, but human beings as such are intentionally related to their world. Where Husserl describes consciousness as intending its object, i.e. as being intentionally oriented towards its object, existential phenomenologists describe human being itself as intentionally oriented towards space and time. Human being means being-in-the-world. That essential directedness of human being to the world, that 'openness' to the world, is intentionality. Thus, Edie says of Heidegger and Merleau-Ponty that 'they clearly agree on the unitary character of "human reality" as a world-directed, active intentionality in whose experience the world is constituted as the human life-world'.[41]

In existentialist terms, then, intentionality is the radical interdependence of subject and world. Again, it is not to be seen as *identification* with the world. Subject and world are to be distinguished. While subjects interact with the world, they also stand back from it, questioning it and wondering at it, and the objects are not only acted upon by subjects but are also resistant to such action.[42] Nevertheless, there is union — communion, even — between subjects and their world. Merleau-Ponty speaks of 'natal bonding between me who perceives and what I perceive'.[43]

What intentionality means is that human experience always points to something beyond itself. It is essentially related to the phenomenon — to the object of experience, to *what* is experienced. As Merleau-Ponty has stressed,[44] phenomenology explores the mystery and paradox of experience: that something which is strange and 'other' is yet able to enter one's consciousness and become part of it. Phenomenology is not about isolated subjects.

Accordingly, because of the essential relationship which experience bears to its object, phenomenologists believe that experience cannot be adequately described in isolation from its object. In their view, experiences cannot be understood to constitute a separate sphere of reality which is subjective and stands in contrast to the objective realm of the external world. To them, such a dichotomy between the subjective and the objective is untenable. Subject and object, distinguishable as they are, are always united. It is that insight which is captured in the term 'intentionality'.

Consciousness: Milieu of the universe

For phenomenology, intentionality is of the essence.

This is the case with the first phenomenologists. Husserl describes intentionality as 'the general theme of "objectively" oriented phenomenology' and 'a concept which at the threshold of phenomenology is quite indispensable as a starting-point and basis'.[45]

It is the same with Heidegger, as Calvin Schrag observes:

> Heidegger is at one with Brentano and Husserl in his view that intentionality is the presupposition of the phenomenological method. In his *Ideen* Husserl made the notion of intentionality a fundamental theme of his philosophy ... Heidegger follows Husserl in his accentuation of the theme of intentionality.[46]

Later phenomenologists continue this emphasis. We find Natanson describing intentionality as 'the axis of phenomenology',[47] while Ainlay asserts its 'undeniable centrality to phenomenology', claiming that 'the initial intent of placing intentionality at the nexus of the phenomenological approach was to save it from the errors of both dogmatic objectivism and subjectivism'.[48]

Despite this centrality, and despite the fact that each of the thirty pieces of nursing research analysed in the previous chapter claims to be phenomenological in approach or to be using the phenomenological method, the word 'intentionality' occurs in them only once. Even in that one instance the word is not used to explain phenomenology, nor is it used in its phenomenological sense. Diekelmann[49] is discussing some unfortunate outcomes of testing and evaluation in nursing education. Insisting that teachers do not 'intend' these outcomes, i.e. have not 'desired' them, she adds facetiously, 'Intentionality is not the issue here!' This is to psychologise the notion of intentionality and understand it in a voluntarist sense.

This appears typical of the treatment of intentionality, meagre as it is, in the nursing literature. Benner and Wrubel offer a more nuanced but not less psychologised view in their *Primacy of Caring*. They refer to people consciously planning to achieve certain ends and consider this too narrow a view of intentionality.

> It leaves out the precognitive forms of intentionality: meaningful, purposive behavior that is based on skilled practices, habits, and language. This alternative form of intentionality is more basic and pervasive than pure forms of intentionality and makes possible smooth functioning and behavior without elaborate conscious deliberation.[50]

This, unfortunately, still misses the point about intentionality. Intentional, as used in phenomenology, does not mean 'purposive', even if this latter word is taken to include activity carried out without actual deliberation.

Marilyn Ray, also a well known proponent of phenomenology in nursing research, offers an accurate definition of intentionality. She tells us that it is 'essentially a character or a property of acts that is always directed toward an object'. Thus, she says, consciousness is intentional because 'consciousness is always consciousness of something'. So far, so good. Following that, however, Ray goes on to an explanation that can only be taken to embody a voluntarist understanding of intentionality.

> For the clinical nurse or researcher, the intentional activity is directed toward caring for a client or toward uncovering the meaning of the specific caring interaction (the lived experience of nurse and the client).[51]

Here the everyday meaning of 'intention' seems to have taken over. In phenomenology, intentionality does not refer to conscious deliberation, or to goal-oriented behaviour, or even to the purposive activity based on habit or routine. It is an epistemological concept (for some phenomenologists, an ontological concept also) and not a psychological one. It has to do with union of object and subject.

This neglect or misconception of intentionality in the nursing literature should be no surprise. Nursing phenomenology, like other examples of the new phenomenology, is not based on the bringing together of objectivity and subjectivity which intentionality encapsulates. It is concerned essentially with the subjective. Much of the research investigated in Chapter 1 states this explicitly: it is about 'attitudes' or 'feelings' or everyday, individual 'perceptions'. Even where articles talk of phenomena, they generally end by identifying phenomena with subjective experiences and rest content with pointing to subjective experiences as such.

When Anderson, for instance, studies immigrant women experiencing chronic illness, she is seeking to learn how women in chronic illness feel about themselves and what the implications of these feelings might be. She speaks of 'the construction of illness' but she does not explore the structure that chronic illness assumes in their experience of it. She talks of the 'construction of the devalued self' but she does not explore the structure of the devalued self. Instead, she is content to show that these women do feel devalued and to indicate how this feeling of being devalued arises and how it is reinforced, for example, by health providers.

Bennett researches 'adolescent girls' experience of witnessing marital violence'. In the light of the phenomenological approach we have been considering, we might expect something to have been uncovered about what marital violence is, precisely as it is experienced in the lives of these girls. From this study, we learn quite a lot about the girls. It is found, for instance, that they:

- have difficulty recalling specific episodes of violence
- have come to live just from day to day
- feel the impact of marital violence in the form of fear, a sense of helplessness, and a sense of loss
- want above all to get away from the violence
- feel a need to understand why the violence happened
- find ways of coping
- feel a need to resolve or 'settle' the experience by coming to terms with it and achieving a sense that they could deal with abusive behaviour if confronted with it again.

This is most useful material for nurses called upon to assist clients who are or have been in a situation of family violence. It tells us a great deal about clients of this kind. But does it tell us anything about the phenomenon of marital violence itself as the object of these girls' experience? There may well be a starting point for delineating the phenomenon of marital violence in what Bennett reports on the experience of fear, the sense of helplessness and the sense of loss, but this is never the real focus of the study.

In her research, Bowman worked with people experiencing chronic low back pain. Although, for Bowman, the goal of phenomenology is 'to make clear the meaning or essence of the phenomenon under study' and her paper is headed 'The meaning of chronic low back pain', she does not attempt to delineate the structure of the pain as it is experienced. The participants are asked what it is like for them to live with their pain. Bowman's findings have to do with participants experiencing pain and with the associated physical symptoms, psychological reactions and enhanced sensory awareness, rather than with the pain itself as experienced, i.e. the phenomenon of the pain.

Interestingly, Bowman's findings include 'altered daily performance'. This evokes, among other things, the notion of disability as a phenomenon in the lives of these people and offers another possibility for more objective treatment. In relation to this section of the findings Bowman writes instead of the hopelessness which the respondents feel at not being able to work, their concern to meet their financial responsibilities, and their distaste for being on disability allowances or Social Security. This, again, is to approach the issue in a totally subjective manner. Yet there is scope here for phenomenological analysis of the disability they experience. How would they describe disability as a phenomenon that they experience? How does disability present itself in their consciousness? What is its structure within their experience of it? It is possible to address these questions in a phenomenological way, but that would be a different project from what Bowman has embarked upon.

'Desire for control' is also a phenomenon of human experience amenable to phenomenological investigation. This forms the focus of

Montbriand and Laing's paper on 'Alternative health care as a control strategy'. It is an issue, Montbriand and Laing say, that calls for further research. However, the questions raised in this study have to do with whether, in ostensibly desiring control, patients are really desiring to escape being in control, whether patients have a twofold locus-of-control orientation (internal and external, with 'giving away control' perhaps being another way of saying 'operating with an external locus of control'), and whether patients are taking for control what is really only illusion of control. As it happens, these questions derive not from Montbriand and Laing's own study but from the literature. Some of the data are then related to these issues in one way or another. Coming to the data with such preconceived concepts, along with the predetermined issues they raise, would seem to violate the norms of nursing phenomenology itself. In any case, there is no genuine phenomenological inquiry undertaken. There is no attempt to describe 'desire for control' as it appears in the experience of these subjects. This is, once again, is to focus on the subjective rather than the objective, on the noetic rather than the noematic. Phenomenological inquiry — 'intentional analysis' — embraces both.

It is interesting to note how nurse researchers cite Spiegelberg, Colaizzi, Giorgi, van Kaam or van Manen, all of whom place clear emphasis on phenomena, but are able to ignore this emphasis and focus exclusively on the subjective in their actual research analysis. A number of the articles examined in Chapter 1 draw on Carolyn Oiler who, in a work she co-edited with Patricia Munhall[52] offers an excellent account of the aims of the phenomenological method. Oiler states, for example, that the 'first task is to dismiss the notion of subjectivity as referring to personal and highly private phenomena'. 'It is', she tells her readers, 'the perceived world that is studied, not subjective phenomena.'[53] Wolf is one who draws on Oiler. She is describing her research into 'nurses' experiences giving post-mortem care to patients who have donated organs'. 'Phenomenological methods', says Wolf, 'emphasize the importance of the subjective experience', and she cites Munhall and Oiler's publication in support of this statement. Wolf goes on to relate how, in 'semistructured interviews', she put to her subjects a series of questions relating to ...

- the 'impression' which post-mortem care has made on them
- what they are trying to accomplish in post-mortem care
- what they experience before, during and after post-mortem care
- what difference post-mortem care makes within themselves
- what makes the post-mortem care experience easy or difficult, enjoyable or disagreeable
- whether, and how, the experience of giving post-mortem care to organ donors is different from giving post-mortem care to others.

All but the last of these points relate to the experiencing nurse and not to the phenomenon experienced. Here Wolf seems to have overlooked

Oiler's warnings in the work which she has already cited. In that final point Wolf seems at last to be focusing on the phenomenon and drawing near to a phenomenological inquiry. Not that she does so in a very wholehearted fashion. She tends to reason about why the one experience differs from the other rather than letting the difference emerge from describing each of them. The experience of post-mortem care in the case of organ donors is influenced, she tells us, by factors such as ...

- the patient being already brain-dead at the time of the donor surgery
- procurement surgery not being curative, palliative or reconstructive
- the brain-dead patient being kept alive by technological means until organs are procured
- organ procurement surgery being associated with the brain-dead patient's 'final death'
- the gift of organs meaning that part of the brain-dead patient lives in another person.

Still, there is at least a starting point for some real phenomenology here. How do these factors show up in the actual phenomenon of post-mortem nursing care of organ donors? Describing that would be phenomenological enough.

To all this, nurses may well want to reply that the nature and structure of the objects of experience are not the problem. As they see it, what needs to be determined is how people view these objects and how people react to them. After all, chronic illness is defined clearly in every nursing textbook. Nurses have been put down often enough to know what devaluation of self really means. Nor is there a nurse anywhere who does not know the meaning of pain: they have seen it and responded to it more often than most. Yes, there are many forms of disability but surely the meaning of disability is not in question. And, what with medical dominance, hospital bureaucracy and a matron tradition that only too often is alive and well despite Director-of-Nursing nomenclature, who better than the nurse knows the meaning of control or desire for control? Even post-mortem care holds no mysteries. On the other hand, people do hold mysteries. People have different understandings and reactions. Pinning down their highly individual perceptions and responses is where the effort should go.

Intrinsic to this line of thought is the view that, while there are perhaps as many subjective meanings of any object as there are subjects perceiving it, behind them all is an objective meaning that inheres in the object. You perceive a fire and for you it is comforting, a thing of joy. It summons up for you the warmth and security of the family hearth. I perceive a fire and it is loathsome, a cause of great fear, for I am the survivor of a bushfire that cost me my family and my home. But, for all that, it is claimed, a fire is a fire. Objectively, what you encounter and what I encounter are one and the same thing. We know what a fire is. What we need to concentrate on is how you and I perceive fire and react to fire.

To think in this fashion is to share the epistemology of positivism. True enough, nursing phenomenologists who think like this place paramount importance on subjective understanding whereby individuals 'mirror' or 'approximate' objective reality. Positivists, on the other hand, are likely to discount subjective understandings and seek to establish objective meaning instead. The two are at opposite ends of the spectrum. The point is that they accept the same spectrum. And the spectrum is 'objectivism'.

Objectivism, phenomenologists say, stands diametrically opposed to the phenomenological perspective. For them, the notion of meaning independent of mind is unthinkable. It is, indeed, a contradiction. The fire you see and the fire I see are different fires. They have different meanings. There is no such thing as meaning that inheres in an object independently of any subject. There is only meaning *for* someone.

In telling fashion Psathas underlines this essential unity of subject and object:

> Phenomenology does not divide or separate the knowing subject from the object of study in order to concentrate on one or the other. The world is not filled with objects that have appearances independent of humans who experience them, nor does subjective experience exist independently of the objects, events, and activities experienced. There is no pure subjective subject or pure objective object. Phenomenology recognizes that all consciousness is consciousness *of* something (where 'thing' is not to be taken to literally mean an existential object). Intentionality is the term used to refer to this relation.[54]

Phenomenology, then, removes the wedge which objectivist thought has driven between the objective and the subjective. There is no object which, in any meaningful sense, exists apart from a subject. There is no fact which, in any meaningful sense, stands alone, free of interpretation. There is no thing which, in any meaningful sense, exists independently of consciousness. Because of this, it makes sense to seek object in subject, fact in interpretation, thing in consciousness. The 'objectivities', Husserl has told us, are discoverable through making consciousness a theme for inquiry.

Among the nursing phenomenologists, few in any sense set their sights on 'objectivities'. Beck is one. Despite the unclarity commented on in Chapter 1, Beck's purpose is to describe the 'essential structure of a caring student-faculty interaction', the 'phenomenon of health', and the 'fundamental structure of postpartum depression'. While she may need to be more single-minded in pursuing this purpose (after all, she includes the 'consequences' of being cared for within the structure of caring, and lists health-enhancing activities as part of the structure of health itself), she is to this extent obeying the phenomenological injunction to return 'to the things themselves'. Wondolowski's findings can be seen as constituting the phenomenon of health rather than describing the purely subjective. Rose too is looking to the phenomenon: she wants to describe 'inner strength' as it appears in the experience of the women she is working with. This seeking of the object in the subject, as we shall see, is not the only requisite for genuinely phenomenological inquiry but, in this respect at least, these nurse researchers are treading the phenomenological path. Most are not.

Merleau-Ponty expresses this aspect of phenomenology well when he describes phenomenology as an 'inventory of consciousness as milieu of the universe'.[55] We should not be misled by his use of the word 'consciousness' in this context. Here, and in his other references to it, Merleau-Ponty is not taking consciousness in a highly mentalistic sense. For him, as Gillan points out, 'consciousness is not act, but life' and opens 'avenues to the discovery of the being of the world'.[56] Merleau-Ponty understands consciousness from an existentialist perspective that sets it firmly in the context of an embodied being-in-the-world.

> The perceiving mind is an incarnated mind. I have tried, first of all, to re-establish the roots of the mind in its body and in its world.[57]

Even given that understanding, what are we to make of 'consciousness as milieu of the universe'? Like so much of what Merleau-Ponty writes, the statement brings us up short. Milieu of the universe? 'Not the other way round?', we find ourselves asking. Should we not be saying that the universe is the milieu of consciousness? It comes so naturally to us to think of consciousness as located within the world and seeking knowledge of that world. That, of course, is part of the 'natural attitude' which Husserl speaks about so much and which, as we shall see, he wants us to 'bracket'. Phenomenology views things differently and it is that different viewpoint that Merleau-Ponty is expressing. Rather than finding consciousness in the universe, we find the universe in consciousness.

And it is *only* there that we find the universe. Never in human history, and nowhere in the world, has there ever been knowledge of reality that has not come into being in and through consciousness. The reality the world holds for us is located in conscious awareness.

Phenomenology invites me, then, to adopt another 'point of view, namely that of consciousness, through which from the outset a world forms itself around me and begins to exist for me'.[58] This is the phenomenological attitude and, as Bossert points out, it makes a difference to how we view our world:

> The first major change upon adopting the phenomenological attitude is that one no longer just sees things and lives through events in the world; rather, one notices that one is having experiences which are meaningful or 'make sense' and that 'things' and 'events' are the meanings (the sense made) of experience. In other words, things and

47

events as objects in the world, and the world itself as an ultimate horizon of objectivity, are now seen as the sense that has been and is being made of pre-predicative experiences.[59]

This phenomenological attitude is a radically different viewpoint and it does not come easily. As Husserl puts it, phenomenology brings 'a wholly new dimension' to philosophy and calls for 'an entirely new point of departure and an entirely new method'.[60] It is in the light of this new dimension and method that we need to interpret Husserl's catchcry, 'Back to the things themselves', with which this chapter began. The journey back to the things themselves is a return to the objectivities enshrined in human experience itself. In Merleau-Ponty's terms, it means looking to a universe whose milieu is consciousness.

Yet the contents of consciousness do not all have the same status. Not all experiences give us access to what we are after. We need to return to a special class or level of experiences. It is variously described, but one name for it is *immediate* experience.

NOTES

1 Pickles (1985), p. 5. More flippantly, Ricoeur (1967, p. 4) says that 'in a broad sense phenomenology is both the sum of Husserl's work and the heresies issuing from it'.
2 See the entry in Husserl's diary cited in Spiegelberg (1982), p. 76.
3 Husserl (1931), p. 28.
4 In Spiegelberg (1981b), p. 182.
5 Husserl (1970c), p. 2. *Cartesian Meditations*, based on Husserl's 1929 Sorbonne Lectures, appeared in French translation in 1931. The German version was published posthumously.
6 See Sallis (1973).
7 This catchcry of the phenomenological movement is commonly attributed to Husserl. Spiegelberg (1975, p. 15) may be a trifle pedantic in suggesting that the phrase in this precise form does not occur in Husserl's published writings. Husserl does say in *Logical Investigations*, 'We must go back to the things themselves' (1970a, II, p. 252). He also tells us to 'leave the last word to the things themselves' (ibid, I, p. 45). and asks that research start 'not from philosophies but from things and from the problems connected with them' (1965, p. 146).
8 Cited by Spiegelberg (1982), p. 81. Found in *Ideen* III [*Husserliana* V, 75] and repeated by Husserl at the start of his London Lectures in 1922.
9 Spiegelberg (1975), p. 76.
10 Husserl (1970a), Vol.I, pp. 44–45.
11 The perception that Heidegger was the first to set phenomenology in an existentialist context is questionable on two scores. For a start, although he is commonly classed as an existentialist, Heidegger vigorously rejected the label. See the discussion of this in Chapters 3 and 4. Secondly, even if Heidegger is viewed as an existential phenomenologist, it seems that the Spanish philosopher, Ortega y Gasset, had preceded him. 'For the historical record', writes Robert O'Connor (1979. p. 59), 'Ortega was probably the first

phenomenologist to take the existential turn, since he claims to have begun criticizing Husserl and developing this position as early as 1914.'

12 Heidegger (1962), p. 50.
13 See Gorman (1977), p. 145.
14 Kockelmans (1965), p. 18.
15 Spiegelberg (1982), pp. 681–719.
16 Omery (1983, pp. 52–53) literally sets the Spiegelberg outline side by side with the methods of Giorgi and van Kaam. However, Spiegelberg goes to some pains to explain exactly what he means by this account of phenomenological method. Looking back on the phenomenological approach he had first outlined in *The Phenomenological Movement*, Spiegelberg (1975, pp. 56–57) says, 'I tried to distinguish between several steps or phases of the method, arranged largely according to the degree to which they were common ground among all those who identified with the phenomenological movement. Let me call this the staggered approach.' In his preface to the third edition of *The Phenomenological Movement* (1982, p. XLV), Spiegelberg repeats the warning he issued earlier in connection with this outline of phenomenological method: 'I did not mean to suggest that these steps have to be taken in rigid sequence in every concrete phenomenological investigation. They are "steps" only in order of importance and spread.' That Spiegelberg's outline is not intended as a step-by-step plan for any given piece of research is indicated by the fact that the sixth element ('Suspending belief in existence') is seen by Spiegelberg as 'a distinct aid to all the steps'. If these were steps in the sense of actions to be taken in sequence, this would have to be Step 1. Spiegelberg came, in fact, to describe these elements as phenomenologies rather than steps. Omery (1983, p. 51) refers to one such listing on his part (descriptive phenomenology, phenomenology of essences, phenomenology of appearances, constitutive phenomenology, reductive phenomenology, hermeneutic phenomenology) but her statement that 'Spiegelberg has identified the six steps of the method that are common to all interpretations and modifications of phenomenological philosophy' is unfortunately worded.
17 Spiegelberg (1982), p. 689.
18 *Ibid.*, p. 688.
19 van Kaam (1966), p. 295.
20 Rose is the only one of the thirty researchers examined in Chapter 1 to suggest anything similar. She states that participants were selected for the study 'if they met Colaizzi's criteria of being able to acknowledge that they have the lived experience of a specified phenomenon and of being able to articulate their experience as they live it in their daily life'. See Rose (1990), p. 59.
21 van Kaam (1966), pp. 317–321.
22 Giorgi ((1970), pp. 134, 139.
23 van Manen (1990), pp. 62–63.
24 See Moustakas (1961). Moustakas distinguishes his method from features which he understands to be characteristic of phenomenological research (see Douglass and Moustakas 1985, p. 43). However, none of these features are necessary to the phenomenological approach and his own study proceeds along unmistakably phenomenological lines.
25 Moustakas (1981), pp. 210–211, 213.
26 *Ibid.*, p. 213.
27 *Ibid.*, p. 214.
28 Thévenaz (1962), pp. 90–91.
29 Bochenski (1974), p. 135.
30 *Ibid.*, p. 136.

31 Brentano (1973), p. xv.
32 In Spiegelberg (1981b), p. 183. The word order in this quotation has been slightly altered to make it more easily readable.
33 This appears as 'inexistence' in the text, although it appears in hyphenated form in the following paragraph. It is hyphenated because Brentano's 'inexistence' has misled some of his readers into thinking that he means non-existence. Brentano means 'existence in', an 'indwelling'.
34 Brentano (1973), p. 88–89.
35 Weinberg (1959), p. 58.
36 See Maritain (1959), p. 112. Here the distinguished French Thomist, Jacques Maritain, expounds the teaching of John of St Thomas on this point.
37 This rejection by phenomenology of the Kantian distinction between *phenomena* and *noumena* has escaped a number of nursing phenomenologists. 'Phenomenology,' say Gortner and Schultz (1988, p. 22), 'is "the study of phenomena, the appearance of things ... as opposed to *noumena*, the things themselves".' Here they are citing Cohen (1987, p. 31), as do Baker, Wuest and Stern (1992, p. 1356) also.
38 Gurwitsch (1967), p. 118–119.
39 Pickles (1985), p. 17.
40 Husserl (1981), p. 15.
41 Edie (1964), p. xviii.
42 See Hammond et al. (1991), p. 97.
43 Merleau-Ponty (1968), p. 32.
44 See Merleau-Ponty (1964a), pp. 92–97.
45 Husserl (1931), pp. 241, 245.
46 Schrag (1967), pp. 280–281.
47 Natanson (1973a), p. 103.
48 Ainlay (1983), p. 4.
49 See Diekelmann (1992), p. 75.
50 Benner and Wrubel (1989), p. 54.
51 Ray (1985), p. 89.
52 See Munhall and Oiler (1986).
53 Oiler (1986), pp. 70–71.
54 Psathas (1973), p. 14.
55 Merleau-Ponty (1965), p. 199.
56 Gillan (1973), p. 6.
57 Merleau-Ponty (1964c), p. 3. For Merleau-Ponty, Kaelin observes (1962, p. 369), 'philosophical reflection is based ultimately upon the lived experience of a "body proper". Consciousness is of an object because a consciousness is not distinct from the corporeal nature of man which already enjoys physical commerce with the objects of the real world.'
58 Merleau-Ponty (1962), p. ix.
59 Bossert (1985), p. 55.
60 Husserl (1964), p. 19.

3

Immediate experience

Phenomenologists, in insisting that we return 'to the things themselves', are telling us to be guided by experience and not by taken-for-granted concepts or inherited principles. In saying this, they rather sound like empiricists. This is the case whether we take empiricism to mean the use of methods based on practical experience rather than some accepted body of theory (its ordinary sense) or the theory that all knowledge derives from experience (its more philosophical sense).[1]

We have noted how Brentano described his psychology as empirical, his best known work being *Psychology from an Empirical Standpoint*. With Husserl's approval, Eugen Fink, who was his assistant from 1930 until his death in 1938, described phenomenology as a 'radical empiricism'. Max Scheler (1874–1928), an early (if unorthodox) follower of Husserl, also liked to describe phenomenology in such terms, calling it 'the most radical empiricism and positivism ever developed'. Even Husserl was content to have his position likened to that of the positivists:

> If by '*Positivism*' we are to mean the absolute unbiased grounding of all science on what is 'positive', i.e., on what can be primordially apprehended, then it is *we* who are the genuine positivists.[2]

In similar vein, Merleau-Ponty considered his philosophy a 'phenomenological positivism which bases the possible on the real'.[3]

There are, of course, basic differences between phenomenology and what the history of philosophy knows as empiricism. For one thing, traditional empiricism tends to restrict genuine knowledge to that of individual physical things. Moreover, for many empiricists it is sense-data that constitute the full gamut of certain knowledge. This is far too limited a viewpoint for phenomenology, which looks to experience as the source of knowledge but has a broad and very rich concept of what experience is. So we find phenomenologists admitting as experience, and therefore as the source of valid knowledge, a whole range of phenomena that are rejected by empiricists.

At the same time, phenomenologists do discriminate among experiences, with one kind being accorded special status as 'phenomena'. Phenomenologists have various ways of addressing these privileged phenomena. We can start with Husserl.

The phenomenal field

Husserl relates valid knowledge to its 'ultimate sources ... principles seen authentically and understood as insights ... whatever is clearly seen, which thus constitutes the 'original', or what precedes all theories, or what sets the ultimate norm'.[4] He tells us that *'whatever presents itself in "intuition" in primordial form* (as it were in its bodily reality), *is simply to be accepted as it gives itself out to be'*.[5] What characterises these ultimate sources or principles, these original, pretheoretical phenomena, is 'the self-evident givenness of individual objects of experience, i.e. their pre-predicative givenness'.[6]

There are several points to note about these statements by Husserl.

First, he is pointing to 'ultimate', 'original', 'primordial' phenomena that 'give' or 'present' themselves to our consciousness in a 'prepredicative' way, i.e. before we engage in any reasoning about them. That rules out introspection, at least in the usual sense of the word. There is no induction or deduction. Within the field of primordial phenomena, says Kockelmans,[7] 'Husserl does not want any induction or deduction but solely intuition on the basis of a very exact analysis and description.' (So, when nurse researchers Beck[8] and Omery[9] refer to phenomenology as 'an inductive, descriptive research method', they are talking about a project that is different from Husserl's.)

Hence the second point to be noted: we grasp these fundamental phenomena not by rational processes of this kind but by 'intuition'.

And, thirdly, what we grasp are 'insights': we see them 'authentically'; they are 'self-evident'; such an insight is 'simply to be accepted as it gives itself out to be'.

Kockelmans sums this up:

Husserl does not see the ultimate root, the radical and absolute starting point of philosophy, in any single basic concept, in any single fundamental principle, in one simple cogito, but in an entire field of original experiences. His philosophy is a phenomenology precisely because it has as its starting point a field of primordial phenomena ... None of the methods used by other sciences can be of value here, because they have to presuppose something in addition to what is actually given, while in the field of primordial phenomena presuppositions are simply inconceivable.[10]

This same understanding of phenomenology as a return to ultimate sources that are self-evidently given to consciousness is found in Husserl's early disciple, Johannes Daubert. Daubert was a student of Theodor Lipps in Munich. In 1902, after reading Husserl's *Logische Untersuchungen*, Daubert cycled from Munich to Göttingen to talk with Husserl. The outcome was a visit by Husserl to a group of Lipps' students in Munich and the establishment of the Munich Phenomenological Circle. This forum for discussion of phenomenology led to the formation of a similar circle in Göttingen with a number of students shuttling between the two. This was the birth of the phenomenological movement.

Husserl seems to have placed great confidence in Daubert as a faithful exponent of phenomenology. Husserl's views are echoed in this extract from one of Daubert's manuscripts:

> *Phenomenological reflection* upon the thing starts from givenness: the colors, forms, and the unifying relations between them. Thereby it will not simply restate the popular view, but makes comparisons and asks for legitimacy to bestow on determinate facts it has in mind these or those determinations. In the answers to these questions about legitimacy, in these demands, a determinate objective world, the world pertaining to the senses as it surrounds us, becomes constituted. This is a totally pure and presuppositionless reflection upon givenness and the phenomena that hover before us and that we are unambiguously aware of in perceiving and thinking.[11]

We find the same emphasis in the language used by later phenomenologists. For them too, the prime target of phenomenological analysis is 'primordial phenomena',[12] the 'immediate, original data of our consciousness',[13] the 'phenomena in their unmediated and originary manifestation to consciousness'.[14] We look for these phenomena in our 'immediate experience',[15] in 'the most immediate types of experience'.[16] The phenomena 'present themselves in immediate experience'.[17] They 'appear in the subject's consciousness'.[18] They are 'given in immediate experience, in one's own consciousness of those things'.[19]

What is meant by 'immediate', 'original', 'primordial'? It means that the experience referred to has not been subjected to self-conscious rational processes. It is not our experience after we have developed or applied ways of understanding and explaining it. It is experience as it is before we have thought about it. It is 'prereflective'.[20] It is the 'pretheoretical awareness whereby the ego "lives its experiences" without articulating about or reflecting on them ... the prepredicative processes in everyday life that make predicative experience possible'.[21]

The things and events of our everyday life, Bossert has told us in a passage already cited, turn out to be 'meanings', the sense we have made of our experience. That experience, Bossert goes on to tell us, is prepredicative experience.

 In other words, things and events as objects in the world, and the world itself as an ultimate horizon of objectivity, are now seen as the sense that has been and is being made of pre-predicative experiences ...

By 'prepredicative experience' I understand the raw data of 'givens' in the flow or stream of pure consciousness, ie, that which is available or presents itself in consciousness prior to the processes of objectification (the constitution or making sense of these 'givens' as things and events) and subjectification (the constitution or making sense of these 'givens' as personal experiences of 'mine').[22]

It is to such prepredicative experience — to Merleau-Ponty's 'direct and primitive contact with the world' — that phenomenology asks us to return. The world with which such contact is made is a world that is prior to any formulated knowledge of it.

To return to things themselves is to return to that world which precedes knowledge, of which knowledge always speaks, and in relation to which every scientific schematization is an abstract and derivative sign-language, as is geography in relation to the countryside in which we have learnt beforehand what a forest, a prairie or a river is.[23]

What Merleau-Ponty is talking of here is

... another kind of thought, that which grasps its object as it comes into being and as it appears to the person experiencing it with the atmosphere of meaning thus surrounding it, and which tries to infiltrate into that atmosphere in order to discover, behind scattered facts and symptoms, the subject's whole being, when he is normal, or the basic disturbance, when he is a patient.[24]

Moustakas has this 'kind of thought' in mind when he articulates the aim of his study of loneliness. He set out, he tells us, to discover the meaning of loneliness 'in its simplest terms', desiring to perceive the experience of being lonely 'in its absolutely native state'.[25]

Ortega y Gasset has another way of putting this.[26] Where Daubert talks of starting with givenness and Merleau-Ponty talks of grasping the object as it comes into being and Moustakas talks of perceiving the object in its absolutely native state, Ortega talks of unmasking the thing itself in its very selfhood. The world is a constant carnival, he tells us, and we are surrounded by masks. The mask he is referring to is 'what has to do with a thing' but is not the thing itself. We may want to determine, say, the phenomenon of 'thinking'. When we begin our inquiry, what we encounter are ideas that have to do with thinking ('a swarm of things that pretend to be thinking but are not'). What are these ideas that masquerade as 'thinking' itself? They are, Ortega tells us, the psychological concepts we relate to intellectual activities, the features we see as characterising logical thought, and — a 'denser' mask than the others — the notion of cognition we have come to identify with thinking. These concepts, which have to do with thinking but are not thinking itself, Ortega sees as 'screens' that hide the phenomenon of thinking from us. The masks must be taken off. The screens need to be removed. 'To make patent what is hidden', he writes, 'we must discover, un-veil, de-nude it. And when the thing lies naked before us, we say that we behold the truth.'

Quite clearly, what phenomenologists are targeting is not the everyday, taken-for-granted assumptions and understandings of people. It is precisely these everyday, 'commonsense' presuppositions and preconceptions — the 'natural attitude', Husserl likes to style them — that phenomenology calls upon us to set aside. We need to move from common sense to prereflection, from predication to prepredication, from the taken-for-granted to the immediate and primordial.

At this point, it may be helpful to recall the nursing phenomenology discussed in Chapter 1. Nursing phenomenology, as illustrated in the pieces of research analysed in that chapter, is oriented to experiences that are 'subjective' and 'everyday'. We have already seen that the way in which it tends to focus on the subjective, rather than on the objectivity to be found in the subjective, marks it off from mainstream phenomenology. Now the same can be said of its focus on the mundane — on 'everyday' experience. By and large there is no attempt to get behind the mundane to the immediate experience that the phenomenologists talk about so much.

Among the researchers studied in Chapter 1 are two apparent exceptions.

Beck, in one of her articles,[27] defines lived experience as 'how a person immediately experiences the world prereflectively (Husserl, 1970)'. She goes on to explain that she chose the phenomenological method so as to 'understand how women experience postpartum depression prereflectively without classifying or categorizing it into signs and symptoms'. After these promising statements, one looks in vain for an account of how participants were encouraged or helped to get in touch with their prereflective experience. In fact, that is clearly not the purpose of the study. What the mothers are asked to describe is 'postpartum depression as it is experienced in everyday life'. The effort made to refrain from classifying and categorising, it turns out, is on the part of the researcher, not the respondents. Citing Oiler, Beck defines bracketing as a process 'of peeling away the layers of interpretation so the phenomena can be seen as they are, not as they are reflected through preconceptions'. What is left from such a process is 'the perceived world prior to interpretation and explanation'. This is an unexceptionable account of bracketing but, unfortunately, Beck has the researcher doing the bracketing, not the respondent.

> Researchers must reawaken their own presuppositions and make them appear by abstaining from them for a moment (Merleau-Ponty, 1956) ... Prior to each interview the researcher attempted to bracket her experiential knowledge in order to capture the reality outside herself (Swanson-Kauffman & Schonwald, 1988) and to portray accurately the reality described by the mothers who participated in the study.[28]

Rose is closer to the mark. She says that, in her study, 'participants were asked to set aside personal theorizations of the concept and to describe inner strength only as it manifested in their lives'.[29] Although that is no easy thing to do, no express effort seems to have been made to help the respondents to do it. and 'personal theorizations' are not absent from the data reported. Moreover, in the previous sentence Rose has identified the participants' 'lived experience' with their 'feelings. thoughts and perceptions'. Still, in asking her participants to set aside personal theorisations, Rose, as a nursing phenomenologist, is showing a rare awareness — if we are talking of the thirty pieces of research selected for analysis in this study, a unique awareness — that the focus should lie with what 'manifests' itself in experience rather than with what the subject has made of it.

Such an awareness is clearly characteristic of mainstream phenomenology. Its emphasis, as we have seen, is on phenomena as they 'come into being', i.e. as they 'appear' to the subject, 'manifest' themselves to the subject, and 'give' themselves to the subject. One aims at 'seeing the clear apprehension of evident givenness'.[30] In this way mainstream phenomenology emphasises the need for openness to phenomena as they give themselves to the experiencing subject.

Not so the new phenomenology which nurse researchers by and large have espoused. As some of these researchers have expressly stated, phenomena are 'synthesised' or 'elaborated'. This synthesis or elaboration is achieved via a two-step process. First, when they have put together the data gleaned from the subjects' accounts of their individual experience, researchers identify the themes emerging from the data. These themes subsume the commonalities to be perceived within the overall data. In the second step of the process, the themes come together to form an 'exhaustive description', a 'general-level description', or a 'constitutive pattern'. It is this description or pattern that tends to be regarded as the 'phenomenon' and the 'essence' of the experience.

In these terms, the phenomenon must be seen as a construct created by the researcher. This contrasts with mainstream phenomenology in which the phenomenon is not constructed but intuited (and therefore grasped first and foremost, it must be noted, by the subject and not by a third party, whether a researcher or anyone else). Merleau-Ponty states it succinctly: 'The real has to be described, not constructed or formed.' The 'real' for Merleau-Ponty ('the world which is given to the subject') is the phenomenon. It is what gives itself to the subject at first hand, before the subject engages in reflection or reasoning or theorising or talking about it. 'It does not await our judgement', Merleau-Ponty tells us.[31] If we want the real, if we are in search of the phenomenon, we should look to what is given to us immediately in experience and not merely to everyday accounts of experience. Natanson makes this clear:

> The phenomenological attitude, I am saying, is in search of a language adequate to the comprehension of the phenomenon and not phenomena yielded, in a secondary manner, through what is said. Relinquishing the former in favor of the latter, turning to what is said instead of the originary givenness which occasioned the saying, represents, from the phenomenological standpoint, experiential refusal.[32]

It has to be said that the new phenomenology does seek phenomena, in Natanson's terms, 'in a secondary manner, through what is said'. As nurse researchers considered in Chapter 1 have explicitly stated, we discover phenomena through people's descriptions of their everyday, subjective experiences. Phenomena are synthesised or fabricated from everyday accounts.

Far from looking to such accounts, mainstream phenomenology seeks a re-encounter with the phenomena themselves where they alone can be found — in life. It bids us, Merleau-Ponty writes, 'to return to the world of actual experience'. As he goes on to tell us: 'Experience of phenomena ... is the making explicit or bringing to light of the prescientific life of consciousness.' This is not the kind of reflection found embedded in everyday accounts. It is much more. It is a reflection that 'knows itself as reflection-on-an-unreflective-experience' and it changes the very structure of our existence.[33]

Grasping the phenomena in this way is not an exercise in reasoning. As we have already noted, it is not deduction or induction. Nor is it introspection. As Brentano points out, introspection is inner observation, whereas what we are talking about here is an inner *perception*.[34] Instead, grasping the phenomena is an intuitive process that enables us, as we explore the phenomenal field of our lived existence, to grasp the essential structures of the phenomena that present themselves to us, i.e. 'the constitutive structures which make them what they are'.[35]

Up to this point the terminology of phenomenologists has been reasonably consistent and cohesive. It should be noted, nonetheless, that this convergence in language masks significant divergence in meaning. Phenomenologists are not all at one on what they consider the return to immediate experience actually achieves. Some of this divergence needs to be examined. Once again, let us start with Husserl.

Husserl: Towards transcendentalism

What, for Husserl, does the return to immediate experience accomplish? That rather depends on which Husserl one is talking of. Saying that is not as facetious as it sounds. In a letter written in 1930, Husserl reflected on the changes in his thought. He suggested that, while for most people 'Husserl is Husserl', he regarded himself as becoming a different person over the years.

> Every independent thinker would really have to change his name after every decade, since he then has become another.[36]

Husserl's thought developed in distinct phases. He was over forty years of age and had behind him some thirteen years of teaching at the University of Halle before he first moved in the direction of phenomenology. Then an associate professor at the University of Göttingen, where he taught from 1900 to 1916, he first used the word in print in Volume I of his *Logische Untersuchungen* (Logical Investigations). It occurs in a footnote towards the end of that volume, which appeared in 1900 and dealt principally with the foundations of mathematics and logic. While at Halle, his earlier works had to do with the philosophy of mathematics, an interest that led him into the field of logic. Here in Volume I of *Logische Untersuchungen*, Husserl called for a reflective analysis of consciousness to establish the foundations he was seeking. He called this analysis descriptive phenomenology and claimed that it would provide a basis, albeit in markedly different ways, both for empirical psychology and for the critique of knowledge.

It was this phenomenological critique of knowledge that was to shape the rest of his intellectual life. Volume II of *Logische Untersuchungen* was subtitled 'Investigations concerning the phenomenology and theory of knowledge', and it contained, he was later to say, 'genuinely executed fundamental work on the immediately envisaged and seized things themselves'.[37] Volume I had prepared the way for the analyses described in this volume, which ushered in the first phase of Husserl's phenomenology. This phase lasted until his lecture series on 'The idea of phenomenology' in 1906–07 (published posthumously under that title in 1950).

By 1907 Husserl's all-but-exclusive focus on mathematics and logic had waned and he was seeing as 'fair game' for his analysis the full range of phenomena that appear in consciousness. Even now, his primary interest was not in real-life, individual, existing things but in realities as ideal as the concepts of 'number' and 'angle' and 'surface' had been in his earlier studies. What he wanted to grasp, above all, was the essential, not the factual. He was in search of the pure essence that makes experience of any kind possible. This, he believed, is given to us in immediate experience and, if we can get back to that immediate experience, we can take hold on it by a kind of intuition or insight.

How, then, are we to get back to immediate experience? Obviously, we need in some way to abandon the 'natural attitude' that imposes its meanings and understandings on what we experience. It is at this point that Husserl introduces what he here calls the 'epistemological reduction'.[38] When a metal is reduced, it is separated from non-metallic substances. Reduction is a process of purification. What Husserl wishes to bring about is a purification of our consciousness from the dross of the natural attitude and it comes about by a suspension of our belief in the actual existence of the objects of experience. In the natural attitude we accept those objects as existing independently of our consciousness in a real world in which we ourselves exist alongside them. In that real world, according to the natural attitude, the objects — and ourselves — can be studied and valid knowledge about them attained. This is what Husserl calls objectivism, even 'naive' objectivism, and it is a view of things that needs to be laid aside or bracketed. 'Bracketing' is a term, obviously, that Husserl is taking from mathematics. Another term he uses, borrowed this time from the ancient Sceptics, is 'epoché'. The terms are interchangeable and refer to the process whereby Husserl sees the reduction of consciousness being achieved.

In nursing phenomenology, as we have seen, there is frequent mention of bracketing. Whether it is invoked by name or its process simply described, it is regularly presented as one of the distinguishing features, if not *the* distinguishing feature, of phenomenological method. Sometimes there is a specific reference to Husserl. For the nurse researchers, however, bracketing clearly does not mean what it means for Husserl, i.e. suspending the natural attitude. The natural attitude, as Husserl depicts it, postulates the independent existence of the objects of attention. Rather than attempting to put this natural attitude in abeyance, the intention of the nurse researchers is to explore the natural attitude of their subjects as faithfully as possible.

When nursing phenomenology talks of bracketing or the process it is taken to imply, what is said to be suspended or laid aside is the researchers' ideas and assumptions about the information their respondents are providing. For them, the process of bracketing is designed to preclude or at least inhibit the imposing of their own presuppositions and constructions on the data. This is in no way what Husserl is talking about. Through the process of bracketing, he seeks to move from naive understanding of the object to the object itself, understood intuitively, as it presents to consciousness in an original and direct fashion. What the nurse researchers are doing is, in Husserl's terms, laying aside their own 'naive' understandings so as to be open to the 'naive' understandings of their respondents. That, clearly, is a different process for a different purpose. Laudable, to be sure, but different.

In nursing research, as elsewhere, if there is to be bracketing (in the Husserlian sense), people must obviously do their own. Laying aside everyday concepts, judgments and understandings sounds hard enough for any of us to do. It is clearly impossible to do it for someone else or with someone else's data.[39] It is feasible for researchers to help people to do their bracketing and thereby get in touch with their own immediate experience. It would also be feasible for researchers to engage in bracketing in relation to their intersubjective encounters with these participants, for these encounters are themselves phenomena that they, the researchers, are experiencing and might want to describe. But the nurse researchers are not describing the intersubjective encounter. They are describing what their respondents are describing to them. They are bracketing their own presuppositions and preconceptions in relation to the data derived from other people — an admirable initiative but an essentially different exercise from Husserlian bracketing. For Husserl, bracketing is one element in an 'essentially first-person, self-reflective process'.[40]

This first-person, self-reflective process which Husserl invites us to engage in is on his part an attempt to achieve clarity and certitude. His passionate quest for clear and certain foundations continued unabated. It was given expression in 1911 in his well-known article, 'Philosophy as rigorous science'.[41] He was looking for what he termed apodicticity. He wanted the bases of human knowledge to be indubitable, i.e. he sought to exclude not only doubt but the very possibility of doubt. Such a quest has a quixotic ring to it in this post-modernist age but, beginning with his *Ideas: A General Introduction to Pure Phenomenology*,[42] it was to lead Husserl to make more and more of the reduction achieved through bracketing. The reduction came to be known as the phenomenological reduction and, increasingly, as the transcendental reduction.

This latter term offers the concept of bracketing a more positive content than the word itself suggests. It indicates that bracketing, and the reduction it achieves, is not just laying aside mundane understandings but gaining access to the transcendental source of intentional acts. It leads us back to more than just our experience in its immediacy and its primordiality. It leads, Husserl claims, to pure consciousness and the pure Ego.

True enough, each of us is an empirical ego existing in this world and belonging to this world. This is what Husserl refers to as the 'worldly ego' or 'natural human ego'. When we bracket the existence of the world and achieve the phenomenological reduction, we leave the empirical ego behind, along with the world to which it belongs, and the transcendental Ego emerges. The meaningful world we experience presupposes such an Ego. It cannot exist as a meaningful world without such an Ego. In short, the transcendental Ego has a meaning-bestowing role. Husserl goes so far as to claim that it *constitutes* the world as a world that bears meaning. This is the transcendental phenomenology that Husserl continues to wrestle with and develop throughout his remaining years at Göttingen, the period he spent at Freiburg (1916–28), and the years of retirement until his death in 1938. It is now a phenomenology that seeks a secure foundation for knowledge by plumbing the depths of our own subjectivity. This, Husserl says, is a transcendental subjectivity:

> In other words, we understand ourselves ... as *transcendental subjectivity* where by 'transcendental' nothing more is to be understood than a regressive inquiry concerning the ultimate source of all cognitive formation.[43]

When we bracket the world in the way Husserl wants us to bracket it, we are left with two things. One of them is the pure Ego. The other is what Husserl describes by the Latin word *cogitationes*. These are our conscious acts or experiences and they can now be described in a way that does not assume the existence of an external, independent world. Husserl wants us to transcend the life of mundane experience. We move beyond this life of mundane experience by bracketing — or, to use yet another synonym, one which comes to the fore in Husserl's *Cartesian Meditations*, by 'meditating'.

> If I put myself above all this life and refrain from doing any believing that takes 'the' world straightforwardly as existing — if I direct my regard exclusively to this life itself, as consciousness *of* 'the' world — I thereby acquire myself as the pure ego, with the pure streams of my *cogitationes*.[44]

Within these *cogitationes*, i.e. among the conscious experiences that survive the bracketing process, Husserl recognises cognitions that are 'first in themselves and support the whole storied edifice of universal knowledge'. They bear, he asserts, 'the stamp of fitness for this function, in that they are recognizable as preceding all other imaginable evidences'.[45] These are revealed through intentional analysis. Based, as the term suggests, on intentionality, such analysis focuses at once on the noetic and noematic dimensions. The emphasis, that is to say, is on both the subjective acts of consciousness and their objects (the phenomena). Such cognitions, 'first in themselves' and recognisable as such, are for Husserl apodictic and adequate. They serve as a fitting foundation for 'rigorous science'.

Husserl's interest here is not with individual phenomena. He is concerned with essences. He is after 'the essential immanent in the particular: the truth of the given'.[46] He wants to determine what it is that makes the phenomenon what it is. So his process includes another kind of reduction — the 'eidetic' reduction, which involves a laying aside of particulars to allow the universal essence to emerge. Husserl proposes a process in which the meditator 'imaginatively varies' the experience under consideration, adding whatever features prove to be imaginable and discarding those that are not. In this way (which, it should be noted, is independent of the existence of the world and of experience in the world), the essential features of a phenomenon are delineated. Husserl explains it in these terms:

> When I keep on meditating, I, as this Ego, find descriptively formulable, intentionally explicatable types ... Perception, the universal type ... has become the pure 'eidos' perception, whose 'ideal' extension is made up of all ideally possible perceptions, as purely phantasiable processes.'[47]

Pure *eidos* perception? Ideally possible perceptions? Purely phantasiable processes? Obviously, Husserl's call to return 'to the things themselves' is now summoning us to more than what we experience, even 'immediately', in our everyday world. Even from this brief and therefore vastly oversimplified presentation of a complex approach to knowledge and reality that developed over a lifetime, it is clear that Husserl's thought has become quite idealistic. In the end, he is willing to accept that designation. 'Carried out with this systematic concreteness', he writes in *Cartesian Meditations*, 'phenomenology is *eo ipso* "*transcendental idealism*", though in a fundamentally and essentially new sense.'[48]

Husserl, it is true, is not an idealist like Berkeley, who found the source of the world in psychological consciousness. For Husserl, what constitutes our world is a transcendental consciousness reached by way of transcendental reduction. He is concerned, he tells us, with 'transcendental subjectivity as the subjectivity that constitutes sense and meaning'.[49] For many commentators this means that Husserl is neither idealist nor realist in any true sense of either word. He very obviously sees the question of the world's 'real' existence as the wrong question to ask. The sense-existence of the world, its existence as a meaningful world, depends on consciousness and that, for Husserl, is all that matters. Whether a world exists in any other sense is for him an irrelevancy and a distraction. For us, Husserl asserts, there is not, and never can be, a world that exists independently of our experience of it.

> The attempt to conceive the universe of true being as something lying outside the universe of possible consciousness, possible knowledge, possible evidence, the two being related merely externally by a rigid law, is nonsensical.[50]

The least one can say is that, if Husserl is described as an idealist, the term needs to be carefully qualified. Dreyfus makes this clear:

> Husserl is no empirical idealist — he does not subscribe to the phenomenalist view that objects are the sum of their appearances —

nor does he hold with the absolute idealists that objects are ultimately mind-dependent. He takes no stance on these metaphysical issues. Rather, in *Ideas* and all subsequent works, he calls himself a trans–cendental idealist, because he holds that mental activity plays an essential role in making reference possible and in determining the sorts of objects to which we can refer.[51]

When all that has been said, it remains true that, for most of those who followed Husserl into phenomenology, his expanding idealism proved a stumbling block. His philosophy came to be seen as a highly individualistic 'egology', despite Husserl's efforts, right to the end, to deal effectively with intersubjectivity. Those thinkers who recognise the essential relatedness of human being, the inescapably social dimension of all human living, tend to see Husserl's understanding as just too idealistic and even Gnostic. Very few have walked — or continued to walk for long — the path he traced for them. During Husserl's lifetime this was a grave disappointment for him and he became more and more isolated as time went on.

All the same, even those phenomenologists who reject Husserl's transcendentalism have drawn direction and rich insights from his work. Because of the respect they pay him and the debt they owe him, some (Merleau-Ponty is among them) have felt constrained to characterise Husserl's transcendentalism as not essential to his approach and method.

Some have seized upon the concept of *Lebenswelt* (lifeworld) which emerges in Husserl's thought during the last decade of his life as an indication that he has abandoned his transcendental idealism. After all, 'lifeworld' has an honest-to-God existentialist ring to it, especially since Husserl's treatment of it is accompanied by more attention to embodiment and historicity than he paid earlier to these aspects of human being. This has led to the claim that, in his last work, *The Crisis of European Sciences and Transcendental Phenomenology*, which invokes the concept of lifeworld extensively, Husserl finally abandons his transcendentalism and seeks his insights from an exploration of the everyday world rather than the transcendental world of the pure Ego.

The claim is not sustainable. For a start, it is hardly credible that Husserl is making such a full about-turn in these circumstances. Husserl's work on the lifeworld is contained in a part of *The Crisis* that was not published in his lifetime. There was no mention of this work until 1940 when Ludwig Landgrebe, Husserl's former assistant, wrote an article that referred to it. Then Merleau-Ponty engaged in discussion of it in his *Phenomenology of Perception*, which was published in 1945. He had come upon Husserl's use of *Lebenswelt* in the manuscripts when visiting the Husserlian archives at Louvain University in 1939.[52] This was all well after Husserl's death in 1938. On the face of it, it is most unlikely that, without anybody noticing, Husserl had abandoned a quest which had stretched over several decades and constituted the one burning ambition of his life.

More than that, a reading of *The Crisis* makes it clear that Husserl is still as transcendentalist as ever. True, he considers the lifeworld to be closer to the phenomena than the world of science, which he sees as an abstraction from the lifeworld. Accordingly, to reach an appropriate starting point for phenomenology, a kind of naturalistic or mundane reduction is required to bring us back to the taken-for-granted understandings of the lifeworld itself. But it is still only the starting point. Husserl goes on to call for his transcendental reduction as the process that will bring us to the pure Ego and the pure phenomena.

While Husserl's transcendentalism remains essential to his phenomenology, it is not the whole of his phenomenology. Even if he adheres to his transcendental form of phenomenology to the end, this need not detract from the enormous value attaching to the non-transcendental form of phenomenology he put forward in his first years at Göttingen. Husserl, let us remember, never jettisons this early form of phenomenological analysis and description. Admittedly, it becomes for him just a preparatory step towards an increasingly idealist goal. It is a form of phenomenology that he knows can never provide the secure, indubitable foundations of knowledge that he seeks with such fervour. In that sense it is for Husserl an inferior phenomenology. It cannot do for him what he wants it to do.

But what if the goals of phenomenology were to change? What if phenomenologists emerge bent on a different pursuit? What if phenomenologists no longer seek apodictic epistemological foundations but are after a way of approaching reality that will help them make sense of their actual existence in this world and address the real-life problems and issues with which that existence confronts them? Could it not be that, contrary to Husserl's experience of it, phenomenology-without-transcendentalism proves capable of all that these later phenomenologists want of it?

That is precisely what happens.

Existential phenomenology

The birth of existential phenomenology, at least self-professed and publicly acknowledged existential phenomenology, may be traced to a trivial incident which Simone de Beauvoir recounts in her autobiography. It took place in 1932 when she and her partner, Jean-Paul Sartre, were out socialising with Raymond Aron. Aron had been studying phenomenology and, at one stage in the conversation, he pointed to his glass and said, 'If you are a phenomenologist, you can talk about this cocktail and make philosophy out of it.' According to de Beauvoir, Sartre 'turned pale with emotion'. That was the very kind of philosophy he had long wanted to develop.[53]

The following year Sartre went to Berlin and studied there for nine months. His work seems to have focused chiefly on Husserl, but he also had an interest in Scheler, Jaspers and Heidegger. When he came back, he recommended to Merleau-Ponty that he read Husserl's *Ideas*. Between them, Sartre and Merleau-Ponty were to be the spearhead of existential phenomenology.

This is not to ignore the contribution of Martin Heidegger. Heidegger's involvement in phenomenology (and his association with Husserl) antedated that of Sartre by close to two decades and most historians of philosophy characterise him as existentialist. However, Heidegger himself forthrightly rejected the existentialist tag. He had an aversion to labelling of any kind, but this label seems to have been particularly unwelcome and in 1946 he explicitly dissociated himself from existentialism as propounded by Sartre. In Heidegger's view, people were treating his philosophy as an existentialist statement because of a misreading of *Being and Time*.

Being and Time (*Sein und Zeit* is its German title) was published in 1927 in the *Jahrbuch für Philosophie und phänomenologische Forschung* (Yearbook for Philosophy and Phenomenological Research). This was the journal which Husserl had established in 1913 at the urging of his students and with the assistance of members of the Phenomenological Circles.

This book reflects Heidegger's lifetime focus on ontology, the study of being. We have noted Husserl's fascination with the mystery of con–sciousness, which he called the 'wonder of all wonders'. Heidegger uses the same phraseology, but for him the mystery to be wondered at is the mystery of being. As human beings, he points out, we experience 'the marvel of all marvels: that what-is *is*'.[54]

As early as 1907 Heidegger discovered the interest that ontology was to hold for him when Conrad Gröber gave him a doctoral dissertation to peruse. Gröber, later Archbishop of Freiburg, had been principal of the St Conrad Residence where Heidegger lived when studying at the Jesuit secondary school in Konstanz. The dissertation was somewhat dated: it had been written about thirty-five years earlier — by Franz Brentano, no less. Its title *Von der mannigfachen Bedeutung des Seienden nach Aristoteles* (On the Manifold Meanings of Being in Aristotle) hardly makes it sound like bed-time reading. Yet it seems to have caught the imagination of the eighteen-year-old Heidegger. As with Husserl's lifelong exploration of consciousness, Heidegger was now launched on a never-ending search for the meaning of being. Twenty years late the quest bore fruit in the pages of *Being and Time*.

In *Being and Time* Heidegger uses human being as his way in to a study of Being itself. In doing so, he gives every appearance of adopting a clear-cut existentialist standpoint. He seems to be addressing the real-life, concrete existence of human beings in time and space. Later, Heidegger was to claim that this was not so. His analyses are existential (*existenzial*) in the sense that they relate to existence at the deeper level of intelligibility, the realm of the underlying structures (the ontological sphere). But they are not existentialist (*existentiell*):[55] they do not relate to the more immediate level of the concrete acts of existence (Heidegger calls this the ontic sphere). The misunderstanding that his interests are truly existentialist stems, some Heideggerian scholars suggest, from the fact that only the first part of *Being and Time* was written and published and even that was incomplete. If the rest of the work had been produced, it would be clear that Being has primacy in Heidegger's thought, that being-in-time-and-space derives from Being and not vice-versa, and that his is no existentialist philosophy.

In addition, it has been suggested that, existentialist or not, Heidegger's use of phenomenology may not have endured. In *Being and Time*, Demske assures us, 'Heidegger's question about being is readily recognizable as a phenomenological one'.[56] In later work, perhaps as a result of increasing alienation from Husserl and Husserl's obvious rejection of the way he is using phenomenology, Heidegger ceases to use the word in his writings apart from a couple of passing references. Spiegelberg, who has carefully traced the development in Heidegger's use of phenomenology, suggests that after *Being and Time* Heidegger moves more and more to the study of texts, especially Greek texts, rather than the investigation of phenomena in any true sense of the word, even his own. Spiegelberg attributes a limited role to phenomenology in Heidegger's thought. 'It never was an integral part of his philosophy', he concludes. 'It was fundamentally nothing but a phase in his development.'[57]

Perhaps, then, Heidegger is neither an existentialist nor a committed phenomenologist. If this is so, there is great irony here, for he ushered in existential phenomenology as a powerful stream within the phenomenological movement. Krell goes so far as to say that existentialism and phenomenology (and, for that matter, deconstruction) are 'unthinkable without him'.[58] That this decisive influence might emanate from a radical misreading of Heidegger is an intriguing thought.

On the other hand, it is possible that Heidegger, in looking back on *Being and Time* and rejecting any existentialist reading of it, is himself reading into the work a stance that he came to adopt in a clear-cut fashion only later in his philosophical development. In this vein, Demske agrees with Rudolf Beerling's hypothesis that *Being and Time* has two sides to it and this 'suggests the possibility of an authentic and inauthentic understanding of the book, perhaps even in Heidegger's own mind'.[59] More of this in Chapter 4.

As for phenomenology, Heidegger himself seems to consider his approach to be phenomenological to the end. In his 1946 'Letter on humanism' he wrote about 'the essential help of phenomenological seeing'.[60] While still maintaining that, for Heidegger, phenomenology has 'lost its priority in the pattern of his thinking', Spiegelberg admits that, in an interview he had with Heidegger in 1953, Heidegger reiterated his rejection of transcendental phenomenology but in no way dissociated himself from the phenomenological movement or repudiated the phenomenological hermeneutics of *Being and Time*.[61]

Ten years after that interview, Heidegger wrote a preface to William Richardson's *Heidegger: Through Phenomenology to Thought*. The original subtitle of the book was to have been '*From* Phenomenology to Thought'. In his preface, Heidegger writes that this title is appropriate if phenomenology is understood as the philosophical position of Edmund Husserl. On the other hand, if phenomenology is taken to mean 'allowing the most proper concern of thought to show itself', the title, he suggested, should read, 'Through Phenomenology to the Thinking of Being'. He also states that his break with Husserl's position is 'on the basis of what to this day I still consider a more faithful adherence to the principle of phenomenology'.[62] This hardly sounds like someone who has rejected phenomenology. It is Richardson's belief that 'Heidegger's perspective from the beginning to the end remains phenomenological'.[63]

What about Spiegelberg's suggestion that in his later works Heidegger ceases to address phenomena in any true sense of the term? Boelen rejects such a claim. Heidegger's move towards texts, Boelen points out, does not mean that he is no longer going to 'the things themselves' or that he has ceased to be a phenomenologist.

> This allegation overlooks the phenomenological historicity of Being. Heidegger approaches these texts not from the viewpoint of linguistics, but rather from the viewpoint of the truth of Being. Being, for Heidegger, is the e-vent (*Geschehen*) of emerging within the primordial dimension of temporality. Being is *geschichtlich*, historical. Heidegger *is* going to 'the first and last thing-itself' (phenomenon) of thought in the Greek texts, namely to Being in its original historical manifestation.[64]

Whether Heidegger is seen as the pioneer of existential phenomenology or as its precursor, it was in France rather than Germany that this stream of the phenomenological movement gained momentum. Jean-Paul Sartre, Gabriel Marcel, Maurice Merleau-Ponty and Paul Ricoeur are the best-known names in this connection.

There is an air of inevitability about this wedding of existentialism with phenomenology. Max Weber's concept of 'elective affinities' comes to mind in this connection. Weber is referring to the process whereby certain ways of thinking and certain groups of people find themselves drawn to each other in the course of history. Existentialists seem to have had an elective affinity for phenomenology, and phenomenologists for existentialism. It is important to distinguish between them. Existentialism and phenomenology are not the same. We have only to think of Edmund Husserl to know that not all phenomenologists are existentialist. And there have been existentialists who were not phenomenologists. Kierkegaard, the pioneer, is one example. Karl Jaspers is another (an interesting case, since he used phenomenology to develop his psychotherapy but refused to incorporate phenomenology into his existentialist philosophy). However, while phenomenology and existentialism are not to be identified, one has to say that they seem made for each other.

What is existentialism? Only a brave person would attempt a definition. Rather than defining it, we might ponder the description that Maurice Friedman offers:

> 'Existentialism' is not a philosophy but a mood embracing a number of disparate philosophies; the differences among them are more basic than the temper which unites them. This temper can best be described as a reaction against the static, the abstract, the purely rational, the merely irrational, in favor of the dynamic and the concrete, personal involvement and 'engagement', action, choice, and commitment, the distinction between 'authentic' and 'inauthentic' existence, and the actual situation of the existential subject as the starting point of thought.[65]

The actual situation of the existential subject as the starting point of thought? That is where phenomenology comes in. As an epistemological stance, phenomenology has been conscripted in the cause of existentialism as ontology and, to the extent one may use the term in the context of existentialism, as philosophical anthropology. It has proved a valuable ally.

But the traffic is not one way. In harness with existentialism, phenomenology itself undergoes a metamorphosis. For a start, as we have already seen, intentionality comes to be interpreted now as a feature of the total human being rather than of consciousness as such. For the existential phenomenologist, human being is being-in-the-world. What intentionality expresses in the existentialist context is the radical interdependence of subject and world or, as many existential phenomenologists like to put it, the subject's 'openness' to the world. Heidegger leads the way in this re-reading of intentionality. If we want to 'make comprehensible the phenomenon occupying us', we must address the task of 'interpreting more radically' the phenomenon of intentionality.[66] The point Heidegger is making is that we do not encounter objects only by way of perception or predication. We encounter objects by virtue of our very being-in-the-world.

Our being-in-the-world, constituted by intentionality, means a bodily presence and an active presence. Existential phenomenology emphasises our embodiment (we are in the world as bodies) and our dynamic relationship with the world (we act upon the world and, in turn, are acted upon).

Merleau-Ponty has much to say about the body. He directs his phenomenological analysis to the bodily dimensions of human existence, seeing each of us a 'body-subject' who is at all times 'situated' in concrete lived experience. In his view, everything human is embodied, including thought and language. So our return to immediate experience may mean not so much a return to primordial cognitions as a return to unformed bodily action that precedes the formed, or to the gesture that precedes clear and decisive thought. Merleau-Ponty's study of the body-subject contrasts with the very cognitive focus found in the analysis offered by the earlier Husserl and goes far beyond the emphasis which Husserl, in his last years, began to lay on bodiliness.

So, if we are in the world as embodied subjects, we are also in the world as active subjects. Existential phenomenology tends to reflect upon action rather than on thoughts and perceptions understood in a highly mentalistic sense. Moreover, the action to which attention is paid comprises day-to-day activities of people in the world, for the existence of these activities is no longer seen as needing to be bracketed in search of a transcendental realm where truth resides. Husserl made much of St Augustine's words, *Noli foras ire, in te redi, in interiore homine habitat veritas.* This is usually translated (in less than gender-inclusive language) as 'Do not go outside, return within yourself, truth inhabits the inner man'. Responding in existentialist (if equally non-inclusive) terms, Merleau-Ponty has this comment to make:

> Truth does not 'inhabit' only 'the inner man', or more accurately, there is no inner man, man is in the world. and only in the world does he know himself. When I return to myself from an excursion into the realm of dogmatic common sense or of science, I find, not a source of intrinsic truth, but a subject destined to be in the world.[67]

Where Husserl invites us to find objectivities in consciousness and sees those objectivities as, in every meaningful sense, constituted by consciousness, the existential phenomenologist like Merleau-Ponty insists that the world is already there. It must, Merleau-Ponty says, be already there, as a world of 'solid structures' and not mere appearances, for the human being, as being-in-the-world, to engage with it. This has implications for our understanding of the nature of phenomenology:

> It is a transcendental philosophy, which places in abeyance the assertions arising out of the natural attitude, the better to understand them; but it is also a philosophy for which the world is always 'already-there', before reflection begins ... and all its efforts are concentrated upon re-achieving a direct and primitive contact with the world, and endowing that contact with a philosophic status.[68]

Note that Merleau-Ponty does not shy away from the word 'trans–cendental'. For him, the word carries no overtones of aspiring to some sphere of pure consciousness. If we put in abeyance the claims inherent in the natural attitude, it is not in order to remove ourselves from the everyday world but simply to take ourselves back to the more immediate manifestations of its phenomena.

For Merleau-Ponty, phenomenology is a transcendental philosophy because the phenomena it investigates cannot be understood apart from consciousness. This has to be taken as the consciousness of an embodied, ever-active subject, as we have noted earlier. Given that understanding, we find Merleau-Ponty, and existential phenomenology generally, continuing to uphold the pivotal phenomenological standpoint: it is within consciousness, and only within consciousness, that one discovers the world. Phenomenology is a voyage of discovery within that field of consciousness. Merleau-Ponty sums it up:

> In order to indicate both the intimacy of objects to the subject and the presence in them of solid structures which distinguish them from mere appearances, they will be called 'phenomena'; and philosophy, to the extent that it adheres to this theme, becomes a phenomenology, that is, an inventory of consciousness as milieu of the universe.[69]

That world, discovered in consciousness, is no mere invention of consciousness. It is 'already there'. Yet it is not there in the sense in which the everyday realist considers it to be there. While Merleau-Ponty does not claim with Husserl that consciousness constitutes the world, he agrees with Husserl that, for us, there is no meaningful world existing independently of consciousness and waiting, as it were, for us to discover it and grasp its inherent meanings.

Objects in the world are indeterminate, Merleau-Ponty asserts. They do not have clear-cut, inherent meanings. They are paradoxical, in fact. Their determination as objects of this kind or that, as objects with this meaning or that, springs from the interaction of a conscious subject with the world which that subject encounters. If objects have no inbuilt, determined meaning, we may yet say they are rich with potential meanings able to be brought forth by the embodied subject. In unfolding Merleau-Ponty's thought, Ihde speaks of 'a world which is always pregnant with significance, but whose meaning must be rewon through an interrogation of its presence'.[70] Perception, therefore, is neither a discovery of preestablished meaning in the object nor a gratuitous bestowal of meaning on the object. It is a process of dialogue, a dialectic, between subject and object that brings meaning into being for both.

For Ortega y Gasset, too, there is no question of finding meaning simply lying in wait for us. He may speak, as we have seen, of unmasking and unveiling and denuding until 'the thing lies naked before us'. But Ortega is not looking for some kind of Platonic idea or Aristotelian form or Scholastic essence. He is too aware of the dimension of history for that. Meaning is created historically. In trying to take hold of 'thinking itself', for instance, we may reach beyond the screens imposed by our psychological concepts, the formal patterns required by our logic, and the notion of cognition we possess. However, when 'thinking now comes into full view unobscured by the particular forms of which it allows', it is found to be ever at work on such forms, merely 'abandoning yesterday's for those of tomorrow'.

> And that implies nothing less than the fact that every concept claiming to represent human reality carries a date inside or, which is the same, that every concept referring to specifically human life is a function of historical time.[71]

So, when we lay aside our everyday understandings and address the phenomenon that comes into view for us, we do not discover some pure form of meaning. We create, as always, historical forms of meaning. Yet they may well be new meanings. If not, they will at least be renewed meanings. (Natanson, as we saw earlier, talks of an 'enlargement of experience', Thévenaz of the 'deepening' and 'consecration' of our original attitude.)[72] One way or the other, engaging in a sense-creating exercise of this kind — 'interrogating' the world, as Merleau-Ponty would have it, or 'unmasking' the world, to use Ortega's imagery — will challenge very profoundly the inherited and prevailing understandings we have laid aside. Merleau-Ponty confronts us with 'the fact that in order to see the world and grasp it as paradoxical, we must break with our familiar acceptance of it'. When we make that break, engaging in reflection that 'slackens the intentional threads that attach us to the world', we experience the 'unmotivated upsurge of the world' and 'watch the forms of transcendence fly up like sparks from a fire'.[73]

Making that break, experiencing that upsurge and watching those sparks fly is what phenomenology is all about. Once again the contrast with the new phenomenology is obvious. Of the nurse researchers considered in Chapter 1, only Rose appears to have any awareness of the need to lay aside familiar understandings and open oneself to the world in fresh ways.

Yet five of these researchers approach their task avowedly from the perspective of Heideggerian phenomenology. Since Heidegger never fails to point up the importance and value of 'phenomenological seeing', perhaps these five researchers will prove an exception and be found on the side of mainstream phenomenology. We need to look carefully at what they have written.

NOTES

1 See Bedford (1989), p. 88.
2 Husserl (1931), p. 86.
3 Merleau-Ponty (1962), p. xvii.

4   From a draft supplementary preface to the second edition of *Logische Untersuchungen*, cited in Spiegelberg (1982), p. 114.
5   Husserl (1931), p. 92.
6   Husserl (1973), pp. 27.
7   Kockelmans (1967), p. 29.
8   Beck (1991a), p. 19; (1991b), p. 372.
9   Omery (1983), p. 50.
10 Kockelmans (1967), p. 29.
11 Schuhmann (1985), p. 7.
12 Kockelmans (1967), p. 29.
13 Pickles (1985), p. 95.
14 Natanson (1974), p. 8.
15 Psathas (1973), p. 13; Gorman (1977), p. 145.
16 Pickles (1985), pp. 94–95.
17 *Ibid.*, p. 178.
18 Gorman (1977), p. 20.
19 Psathas (1973), p. 13.
20 Rogers (1983), p. 33; Frankl (1968), p. 2.
21 Rogers (1983), pp. 33, 37.
22 Bossert (1985), pp. 55, 65.
23 Merleau-Ponty (1962), p. ix.
24 *Ibid.*, p. 120.
25 Moustakas (1981), p. 210.
26 See Ortega y Gasset (1963), pp. 59–63.
27 See Beck (1992).
28 *Ibid*, p. 167.
29 Rose (1990), p. 60.
30 Kohak (1978), p. 151.
31 Merleau-Ponty (1962), p. x.
32 Natanson (1974), p. 12.
33 Merleau-Ponty (1962), pp. 57, 58, 62.
34 Brentano (1973), p. 29.
35 Schrag (1967), p. 278.
36 From a letter to Georg Misch, cited in Spiegelberg (1982), p. 84.
37 Husserl (1970a), Vol.I, p. 45.
38 The term 'reduction' did not occur in Husserl's *Logische Untersuchungen*, although he added the term when he issued the second edition in 1913. See Smith (1978), p. 434.
39 Ethnomethodologists perform an *epoché* and achieve a reduction not in relation to other people's data but in order to secure that data. 'The ethnomethodologist suspends belief in society as an objective reality, *except* as it appears and is "accomplished" in and through the ordinary everyday activities of members themselves ... Thus, the reduction accomplished here is to bracket the features of everyday life as known to the observer and heretofore understood and accepted by him as he operated in the natural attitude and to consider *as phenomena* only those practices of members which are used by *them* to produce and make regular, consistent, sensible, reproducible, understandable and accountable, *to and for themselves*, the setting's features.' (Psathas 1977, pp. 78, 80) This too, quite clearly, is not the kind of bracketing nursing phenomenologists engage in. Their bracketing does not relate to *what* they look at but to *how* they look at it.
40 Hammond et al. (1991), p. 181.
41 To be found in Husserl (1965).

42 Volume I of *Ideas* was published in 1913. The other two volumes were published posthumously.
43 Husserl (1973), p. 49.
44 Husserl (1970c), p. 21.
45 *Ibid.*, p. 14.
46 Natanson (1973), p. 4.
47 Husserl (1970c), pp. 69–70.
48 *Ibid.*, p. 86.
49 *Ibid.*, p. 84.
50 *Ibid.*
51 Dreyfus (1982), p. 9.
52 See Spiegelberg (1982), p. 144; Hammond et al. (1991), p. 10.
53 See Hammond et al. (1991), p. 1.
54 Heidegger (1949b), p. 355.
55 Translators and commentators have had trouble with *existenzial* and *existentiell*. In their English versions or discussions they have tended to use 'existential' and 'existentiell', respectively, or some variation of these. 'Existentialist' is used here for *existentiell* to avoid the Germanicism of 'existentiell' and because 'existentialist' succeeds in capturing the notion of pertaining to real-life concerns. Admittedly, it has other connotations as well and may have Heidegger turning in his grave, given the vehemence with which he rejected the title of 'existentialist'. Still, there may be consolation in the fact that the word is used here for the issues he says he is *not* primarily concerned with.
56 Demske (1970), p. 12.
57 Spiegelberg (1982), p. 409.
58 Krell (1989), p. 130.
59 Demske (1970), p. 59.
60 Heidegger (1977b), p. 235.
61 Spiegelberg (1982), pp. 406–407.
62 In Richardson (1963), p. XIV.
63 *Ibid.*, footnote.
64 Boelen (1975), p. 113.
65 Friedman (1964), pp. 3–4.
66 Heidegger (1982). pp. 161–162.
67 Merleau-Ponty (1962), p. xi.
68 *Ibid.*, p. vii.
69 Merleau-Ponty (1965), p. 199.
70 Ihde (1973), p. 67.
71 Ortega y Gasset (1963), p. 75.
72 Thévenaz (1962), p. 90.
73 Merleau-Ponty (1962), pp. xiii–xiv. Phenomenology — even Husserl's form of it ('Willy-nilly, against his plans and according to his essential audacity') — 'awakens a wild-flowering world and mind ... This renewal of the world is also mind's renewal, a rediscovery of that brute mind which, untamed by any culture, is asked to create culture anew.' (Merleau-Ponty 1964b, p. 181). According to McCleary (1964, p. xxxi), Merleau-Ponty 'reconfirms the ... need for an untiring phenomenological questioning which seeks to restore the existential encounter between "wild-flowering mind' and "brute being" from which all truth and cultural renewal must and can arise'.

4

The phenomenology of Martin Heidegger

What do the five nurse researchers who claim to be using a Heideggerian approach understand that approach to be?

If we look at what Zerwekh,[1] Watson,[2] Dobbie[3] and Diekelmann[4] have to say, we find them making three principal assertions about Heideggerian phenomenology or hermeneutics. For a start, it is said to be a way of discovering meanings in day-to-day experiences. Secondly, the meanings sought through the Heideggerian approach are not idiosyncratic but 'shared' or 'common'. Thirdly, to discern these meanings, it is necessary to take a holistic view and not divorce people from their context.

None of these understandings attributed to Heideggerian phenomenology adds significantly to the explanation of nursing phenomenology elaborated in Chapter 1. Nor, it has to be said, do these understandings have anything to do essentially with Heidegger's philosophy.

That conclusion, some may want to say, has a decidedly dogmatic ring to it. After all, given the abstruseness of Heidegger's thought, there is plenty of room within Heideggerian scholarship for conflicting interpretations on a broad range of issues. These nurse researchers surely have an unquestionable right to grapple with Heidegger and make their own interpretations of what he is saying. They do, indeed. The problem is that the understandings proffered by these nurse researchers, far from being in any true sense an interpretation of Heidegger's thought, have all the hallmarks of an entirely different provenance. They give no sign of having emerged from interaction with Heidegger's thought and the texts in which it is found. To a large extent, they are diametrically opposed to his intent and method. Let us look again at what these nurse researchers are putting forward. They affirm the everyday subjective experience of individuals. Then, finding this experience embedded in everyday practice and articulated in everyday narratives, they insist on the need to place it within its situated context, i.e. the symbolic meaning-complex which people share as their given culture. In all of this, these researchers can be said to be carrying on the North American intellectual and research tradition of pragmatist philosophy, symbolic interactionism, and humanistic psychology. It is a matter of dressing this tradition in Heideggerian livery rather than a genuine attempt to interpret and apply Heidegger's central notions. And, in the process, the phenomenological character of Heidegger's work is completely lost.

Is it perhaps a question of 'reading against the grain'? It is possible, and surely legitimate (countless people have done it), to engage creatively with the Heideggerian texts in a search for original insights, without direct concern for precise meanings Heidegger may be deemed to have intended in these texts. That would be undoubtedly a valuable way to proceed. There would even be a certain appropriateness about doing that, for Heidegger himself (the early Heidegger at any rate) has something to say about doing 'violence' to texts. The nurse researchers, however, are not claiming to be 'reading against the grain'. They offer their approach, without qualification, as truly Heideggerian in nature. They appear quite clearly to be identifying their approach with what they understand Heidegger himself to be doing.

Here, then, as elsewhere, nurse researchers are substituting a new phenomenology for the phenomenology of the phenomenological movement. It leads them far from the project Heidegger set for himself.

Heidegger's project

In significant ways the fifth researcher referred to is an exception. Marsha Rather[5] takes a different tack. She talks about 'being'. It is the goal of Heideggerian phenomenology, she claims, to reveal 'the nature and meaning of Being'. As humans, we have 'possibilities for being', and grasping these possibilities is what 'understanding' — for us 'a foundational mode of existing' — is all about. Language too is part of the picture: it is a mode of human being which 'unveils Being'.

Rather's discourse brings us much closer to the Heideggerian project. At an early age, as we have already seen, Heidegger was inspired by the writing of Franz Brentano to explore the meaning of Being. The initial letter of the word is capitalised to indicate that what Heidegger is in pursuit of is Being itself. Although Rather tells us that 'Being is the being of whatever is', Heidegger's ultimate interest is not with the 'being of beings'. He criticises traditional metaphysics, and believes metaphysics needs to be 'overcome', because it fails to go beyond the being of individual beings to Being itself. Pöggeler points out how Heidegger, in his best-known work, feels the need to distinguish between Being and beings:

In *Being and Time*, it is stated that 'that which is to be found out by the asking', i.e. the meaning of Being, demands its own manner of being grasped, which manner may not be oriented towards beings ... Metaphysics conceives of beings as beings; it inquires after the Being of beings, but not after Being itself.[6]

Already this is sounding like something very different from what the nurse researchers are engaged with. As they themselves express it, they want to discover 'subjective experience', the wisdom 'embedded in everyday practice stories', the practices and meanings 'embedded in day-to-day lived experiences', or the values and significances which are 'visible' when persons are set in their context. Even for Rather, everyday experience is 'the focus of attention' and 'the concern is to render lived experience intelligible'.

Looking at subjective everyday experience and discerning its visible meanings (or even its 'hidden' or 'implicit' meanings, as Rather would have it), is not what Heidegger is about. Heidegger is after the meaning of Being itself. He is not intent on divining the meanings of real-life experiences. His goal is not to render real-life experiences intelligible in that sense or by that path. While Rather, and countless others, consider the meanings of real-life experiences to be 'possible meanings of Being', this is not the case with Heidegger. To rest content with meaning of that order would be, for him, to fall into the trap in which metaphysics still finds itself enmeshed. It would mean surrendering Being itself for the mere being of beings.

Yet we are talking of the Heidegger who, in *Being and Time*, gives us a profound and impressive analysis of human being (or *Dasein*, to use the term that Heidegger prefers to use).[7] Many have seen in this treatment of human being an existentialist exposition that has led the way for others, such as Sartre and Merleau-Ponty, to follow. Numerous commentators have regarded Sartre's *Being and Nothingness*[6] as, in large measure, a commentary on Heidegger's *Being and Time*. Nevertheless, Heidegger makes it clear that his principal objective, even in this first major work, is to seek the meaning of Being as such. If he focuses on human being — *Dasein* — in *Being and Time*, it is because his true quarry — Being itself — manifests itself there. '*Understanding of Being is itself a definite characteristic of Dasein's Being*', says Heidegger,[9] and he puts these words in italics to emphasise their central importance. In his mind, it is this understanding of Being that distinguishes human beings from 'things'. Because of this understanding of Being as the 'definite characteristic' of *Dasein*'s Being, it is in human being and not in a thing or an idea that, phenomenologically, we find Being manifested. So Heideggerian scholars are quick to point out that in *Being and Time* Heidegger does not centre on human being for its own sake but as the way in to a grasping of Being itself. Boelen, for instance, has this to say:

In order to understand the meaning of Being we have to phen-omenologically rekindle the question of Being. And in order to rekindle the question of Being we have to phenomenologically describe *Dasein* as Being-there, as Being-in-the world, as ex-sistence in the etymological sense of 'standing out', of being an open relation to Being or to totality of all that is.

Now, Heidegger's *Being and Time* is precisely this phenomenological analysis of *Dasein*, of Being-in-the-world, which aims at discovering the fundamental meaning of Being. The existential analysis of *Dasein* in *Being and Time* is not an analysis of man as a human subject, it is not a philosophical psychology or anthropology. The existential analysis of *Da-sein* in *Being and Time* is rather a fundamental ontology of the differentiated self-manifestation of Being-in-the-world.[10]

After *Being and Time*, at least from the time of his *What is Metaphysics?*, there is no doubt at all that Heidegger is dealing primarily and explicitly with the question of Being. From that point on, the phenomenology of *Dasein* slips into the background.

Heidegger, even in *Being and Time*, insists that the task he is setting himself is not 'ontic' (i.e. dealing with 'real life' issues and circumstances, the concrete acts of day-to-day existence) but 'ontological' (i.e. pertaining to a deeper level of intelligibility where the underlying structures of being are to be found). As noted in the previous chapter, he has another way of putting this, at least when dealing with persons: he is concerned with existential (*existenzial*) issues rather than existentialist (*existentiell*) issues. In these terms, he tells us explicitly that the existential definition of concepts must not be accompanied by any existentialist commitments.[11]

There are commentators who, despite Heidegger's protestations, consider his account of human being in *Being and Time* to be inescapably ontic and existentialist. More than that, some maintain, it is a tragic, heroic, pessimistic, even nihilistic, account in the Nietzschean–Kierkegaardian mode. Heidegger may have painted his picture of human being solely to reach forward into Being itself but, such scholars claim, the picture he gives us can stand alone. And, while he clearly sees himself as engaged with ontology and not addressing existentialist concerns, Heidegger comes almost to admit as much when he agrees that there is 'a definite ontical way of taking authentic existence, a factical ideal of *Dasein*, underlying our ontological Interpretation of Dasein's existence'.[12] Nevertheless, he goes on at once to describe this ontic account of *Dasein* as only a 'presupposition' in relation to the theme of his investigation. The presupposition is *Dasein*. The theme is Being.

For Heidegger, *Dasein* is where Being reveals itself — a 'clearing', he likes to say, as in the midst of a dense, dark forest, where Being is lit up and becomes unconcealed. Unlike other beings, humans not only have

Being but have a concern about their Being, an attitude towards Being and some understanding of Being. It is a rudimentary understanding. Heidegger refers to it as 'vague average understanding of Being', an 'obscured or still unillumined understanding of Being'.[13] It is this pre-understanding that must be grasped and unfolded 'with more and more penetration', leading to a grasping and unfolding of that for which it is a presupposition, i.e. Being itself.

Reaching that pre-understanding is already a phenomenology. Its further unfolding, together with the manifestation of Being itself and the unveiling of other phenomena in the light of Being itself, remains a phenomenological process throughout.

> Phenomenology is our way of access to what is to be the theme of ontology, and it is our way of giving it demonstrative precision. *Ontology is possible only as phenomenology.*[14]

For Heidegger, therefore, phenomenology reveals explicitly — in a thematic way — what is already given dimly and implicitly in what he terms the 'fore-structure' of understanding. Here he uses the etymology of the word 'phenomenology' to explain how he understands it. The Greek word φαινόμενον means that which manifests itself. The Greek word λόγος means a speaking forth and therefore 'a making manifest'. Accordingly, phenomenology means making manifest that which manifests itself. This is not as tautological as it may sound at first. As Heidegger puts it, cumbersomely if not tautologically, it is 'to let that which shows itself be seen from itself in the very way in which it shows itself from itself'.[15]

Here Heidegger's phenomenology has a reduction of its own, even if it is not called that. It rejects Husserl's transcendental reduction (one does not bracket existence when one is seeking Being through being) and Husserl's eidetic reduction (Being is not sought as an 'essence' since it is not a genus, Heidegger believes, but transcends the traditional categories). Nevertheless, as we have already seen, Heidegger seeks a phenomenological return 'to the things themselves'. He wants his philosophical inquiry to be rooted in the things themselves and not in 'free-floating constructions' or 'accidental findings' or 'pseudo-questions'.[16] But what are these 'things themselves'? Certainly not day-to-day experiences. Heidegger wants us to reflect on our shadowy pre-understanding of Being, as the prelude to an unfolding of that understanding. We must return to Being itself, revealed by way of *Dasein*. For Heidegger, Being is, and must remain, 'the first and last thing-itself of thought'.[17] If one wishes to use the language of 'reductions', Boelen points out, this is a reduction from naturalistic and cultural prejudices relating to the lifeworld.[18]

'A making manifest of what manifests itself.' That is Heidegger's phenomenology. It is also his hermeneutics.

Hermeneutics

Hermeneutics, Heidegger tells us, 'was familiar to me from my theological studies'[19] The word, which dates from the seventeenth century, is derived from the Greek verb ἑρμηνεύειν, 'to interpret'. In its original use, for a long time its exclusive use, hermeneutics stood for the principles of biblical exegesis. Characteristically, Heidegger takes this word and gives it fresh meaning. In his hands it comes to represent the phenomenological project he has embarked upon.

> ... the meaning of phenomenological description as a method lies in *interpretation*. The λόγος of the phenomenology of Dasein has the character of a ἑρμηνεύειν ... Philosophy is universal phenomenological ontology, and takes its departure from the hermeneutic of Dasein, which, as an analytic of *existence* has made fast the guiding-line for all philosophical inquiry at the point where it *arises* and to which it *returns*.[20]

Here Heidegger is bringing together in a unitary way not only ontology and phenomenology but, through hermeneutics with its connotations of dialectics or rhetoric, the element of language as well. As Richardson puts it:

> ... 'hermeneutics' (the process of letting-be-manifest) and φαινόμενα (that which manifests itself), plus λέγειν (to let-be-manifest), rejoined each other to such an extent that 'hermeneutics' and 'phenomeno-logy' became for Heidegger but one. If 'hermeneutics' retains a nuance of its own, this is the connotation of language.[21]

In this way, starting with a phenomenological return to our being, which presents itself to us in a nebulous and undeveloped fashion, we are invited by Heidegger to 'unfold' that pre-understanding, make explicit what is implicit, and grasp the meaning of Being itself.

This is clearly a different project from the one proposed by the nurse researchers we have been considering — or, for that matter, by the sources they invoke. Diekelmann tells us that 'Heideggerian hermeneutics [was] first introduced to nursing by Benner'.[22] In her many publications relating to nursing research, Patricia Benner has indeed repeatedly invoked Heideggerian hermeneutics. For example:

> The particular kind of hermeneutics the author has used is congruent with a particular theoretical stance (Heideggerian phenomenology) taken toward human beings and human experience ... The kind of hermeneutics described here has it roots in Division I of Heidegger's work [i.e. of *Being and Time*].[23]

In expounding Heideggerian phenomenology, Benner has much interesting material to offer. However, when she comes to the purpose of Heideggerian hermeneutics, Benner is wide of the mark.

The goal is to understand everyday practices and the experiences of health and illness ... The goal is to find exemplars or paradigm cases that embody the meaning of everyday practices.[24]

What has led Benner astray is her notion that Heideggerian phenomenology is 'a particular theoretical stance ... taken toward human beings and human experience'. We need to return to this later, but for the moment we should note that, for Heidegger, phenomenology is a method of philosophising and not any philosophical content.

The expression 'phenomenology' signifies primarily a *methodological conception*. This expression does not characterize the what of the objects of philosophical research as subject-matter, but rather the *how* of that research.[25]

It is not even a method he adopts to explore what it means to be human, in the sense of a philosophical anthropology. Max Scheler may have done precisely that, but that is not Heidegger's interest. Many years after publishing *Being and Time*, Heidegger goes to some pains to disabuse people of that notion:

One need only observe the simple fact that in *Being and Time* the problem is set up outside the sphere of subjectivism — that the entire anthropological problematic is kept at a distance, that the normative issue is emphatically and solely the experience of There-being with a constant eye to the Being question — for it to become strikingly clear that the 'Being' into which *Being and Time* inquired cannot long remain something that the human subject posits. It is rather Being, stamped as Presence by its time-character, that makes the approach to There-being. As a result, even in the initial steps of the Being-question in *Being and Time* thought is called upon to undergo a change whose movement cor-responds with the reversal.[26]

Accordingly, in his hermeneutical project and his use of the phenomenological method, Heidegger's goal is not that of exploring 'meanings of everyday practices'. Instead, he wishes to explore the meaning of Being. If he turns at the start to *Dasein*, to the 'being-there' (or, as this text has it, 'There-being') of humans, it is because *Dasein* constitutes the *locus* where Being is encountered. In short, Heidegger wants it known that, even in *Being and Time*, he is concerned not with the human in the full dimensions of its humanness but with the human simply and solely as *Dasein*, as 'being-there', i.e. as that in which Being manifests itself.

In this passage Heidegger points out something more. He talks of a 'reversal'. The process he describes is one that must soon be turned around. The initial movement may be from *Dasein* to Being but, when that movement is done, Being begins its approach to *Dasein*. The process is circular. As we have noted earlier in this chapter, Heidegger suggests that we make fast the guiding line for all philosophical inquiry 'at the point where it *arises* and to which it *returns*'. We begin with and from a pre-understanding of being — Heidegger's 'fore-structure' — and the task is to unfold that rudimentary understanding, rendering explicit and thematic what is at first implicit and unthematised. This more enlightened understanding of Being then returns to enrich our existence in the world. What Heidegger is alluding to here is his version of the 'hermeneutic circle'. We must, he tells us, 'leap into the "circle", primordially and wholly'.[27]

The term 'hermeneutic circle' has a long history. There is reference to the hermeneutic circle in the writings of Ast and Schleiermacher in the early nineteenth century and later in that century in the work of Wilhelm Dilthey. Heidegger, as one would expect of such an original thinker, proceeds to fill the term with meaning of his own. 'This circle of understanding,' he tells us, 'is not an orbit in which any random kind of knowledge may move; it is the expression of the existential fore-structure of Dasein itself.'[28]

There is reference to the 'hermeneutic circle' in nursing phenomenology too. Rather, for instance, uses the phrase to describe the active participation which the reader of the research report takes in 'the validation process of Heideggerian hermeneutics'. The report, she says, 'intentionally draws the reader into the hermeneutic circle, moving back and forth between excerpts from the data, a Heideggerian analysis of the data, and the emerging description of the constitutive pattern that was unveiled'.[29] Leonard understands the hermeneutic circle differently. She links it to the sharing of culture and language:

> ... all knowledge emanates from persons who are already in the world and seeking to understand other persons who are already in the world. One is thus always within the hermeneutic circle of interpretation. Researcher and research participant are viewed as sharing common practices, skills, interpretations, and everyday practical understanding by virtue of their common culture and language.[30]

Each of these understandings of the hermeneutic circle is useful for its author's purposes (and Leonard's, in particular, relates closely to what Okrent describes as 'the standard sort of *Verstehen* position').[31] Neither understanding, however, can be said to reflect that of Heidegger.

In Heidegger's later works it is the second part of the circle that preoccupies him. There he is concerned directly with Being rather than with *Dasein* as the access to Being. Instead of presenting a phenomenology of *Dasein*, we find him engaging in hermeneutic dialogue with the ancient Greeks, especially the pre-Socratics, and with poets such as Hölderlin.

The early Greeks, Heidegger believes, were in touch with Being in a way that has been subsequently lost. There is an originality about their thought and we need to make 'a painstaking effort to think through still more primally what was primally thought'.[32] This shift in approach — from an analytic of *Dasein* to a running conversation with the early Greek thinkers — reflects a new emphasis on historicity. While commentators detect a certain ahistorical quality in *Being and Time*, the same charge cannot be levelled at the later works. In the course of the 1930s, Heidegger comes to focus more and more on the 'history of being' — the unfolding of Being over time as it gives itself to thought (or withholds itself from thought). Looked at from this perspective, the earliest Greek thought is seen as a 'self-blossoming emergence'.[33] There is a primordiality about it that needs to be recaptured, for there at the dawn of Western civilisation it constitutes a new beginning. For Heidegger, 'the beginning, conceived primally, is Being itself'.[34] Hence his call to think through what is primally thought even more primally.

As for the poets, 'our existence is fundamentally poetic'[35] and Heidegger feels that poetry can lead us to the place where Being reveals itself. It provides the 'clearing' where Being is illuminated. The poet 'reaches out with poetic thought into the foundation and the midst of Being'.[36] The essence of poetry is 'the establishing of being by means of the word'.[37] Thoughtful poetising, says Heidegger, 'is in truth the topology of Being', a topology 'which tells Being the whereabouts of its actual presence'.[38]

Because of this change of direction in the later works — from Being to the human, rather than from the human to Being — commentators have spoken of *die Kehre* (variously translated as the 'turn', 'turning around' or 'reversal'). Heidegger too speaks of *die Kehre*. One of his essays bears that title. However, where many commentators, especially early ones, see the reversal as a 'fundamental change in his thinking',[39] Heidegger himself perceives the reversal as a change in method called for by the very task he is addressing. For him, such reversal is inherent in the circularity of our being and, since he considers understanding a mode of being itself, it is inherent in our understanding too. In his excellent guide for readers of *Being and Time*, Kaelin refers to this circularity:

> This return to an ontic dimension of an ontological 'demonstration', of course, is no accident. For Heidegger, it is required by the nature of an interpretive understanding, as is now clear from the hermeneutical circle we have been traveling.
>
> ... we must remember that understanding is a way for a human being to be; and that our being exhibits a structure that is itself circular: a projection towards a future possibility, but as authentic, resolutely repeating that act which is most our own ... Albeit enriched by the journey, we have only returned to where we were at the beginning of our inquiry.[40]

It needs to be noted that at no point in his hermeneutic circle does Heidegger place the focus on ontic concerns or existentialist interests for their own sake. It is true that he starts his inquiry from the living human being in that human being's real-life context. *Being and Time* and the other early writings are filled with examples drawn from mundane and practical human activities. Heidegger, however, is not looking to elucidate the shared, culture-bound meanings of such activities. As Guignon[41] points out, he is engaging in a phenomenology of everydayness so as to identify the essential structures of any *Dasein* whatsoever. It is a hermeneutic that aims to reveal the primary understanding of the world which he sees as informing all our day-to-day interpretations. The ontic elements, in other words, are explored with the sole aim of moving to the ontological by way of the original pre-understanding of Being inherent in them.

These structures of *Dasein* forming the focus of Heidegger's inquiry he calls 'existentials'. They are structures of being that make human existence and behaviour possible.

Heidegger writes, for example, about 'solicitude'[42] and this certainly comes to be expressed in this-worldly ways. He has already dealt with 'care' or 'being concerned' as an existential structure that emerges once one sets *Dasein* in its context as Being-in-the-world. *Dasein* has to deal with things in the world. At one point in *Being and Time*, Heidegger lists fourteen positive ways and several negative ways in which each of us may relate to entities in our world.[43] This orientation to things, at the level of our being as humans (understood ontologically and not ontically, therefore), Heidegger calls 'care' or 'being concerned'. Care (*Sorge*), as Heidegger uses the word, is a structure of our being and it gets expressed in all the different ways we relate to the entities in our world.

When we are dealing with people and not things, the word he uses is not care or concern but solicitude (*Fürsorge*). Solicitude, Heidegger says, 'corresponds to our use of "concern" as a term for an *existentiale*'. Solicitude is grounded not merely in our Being-in-the-world but in our Being-with, which too is an 'existential'. Our way of being is to be with others and is therefore solicitude. 'Solicitude proves to be a state of Dasein's Being', says Heidegger, and it is expressed in forms such as providing 'food and clothing, and the nursing of the sick body'. In the course of his analysis of solicitude, Heidegger describes the solicitude that 'leaps in' and takes care away from the other. He distinguishes from this the solicitude that 'leaps ahead' of the other, not to take away the other's existentialist potentiality-for-Being, but to 'give it back authentically as such for the first time'. He states that these are 'two extreme possibilities' of the positive modes of solicitude.

In citing this Heideggerian distinction, Benner and Wrubel apply it at once to nursing.[44] In nursing, they tell their readers, 'leaping in' may be unavoidable in cases of extremely ill or dependent patients, but otherwise it is the 'leaping ahead' form of solicitude that commends itself as 'a form of advocacy and facilitation' and a form that 'empowers' others. This

application to nursing of Heidegger's two types of solicitude is useful —
as long as it is remembered that it is Benner and Wrubel's and not
Heidegger's. While Heidegger expressly cites nursing as a form in which
solicitude may be expressed, he makes his distinction between these two
kinds of solicitude for a different purpose from that to which Benner and
Wrubel put it.

In dealing with solicitude, Heidegger has no ethical or pastoral intent.
As always, his purpose is ontological. It is to elucidate the question of
Being. Heidegger is not describing solicitude because it has everyday
meaning and value that is important to people. He is not making his
distinction in order to urge people to 'leap ahead' rather than 'leap in',
even though, as he points out, through 'leaping in' the Other can become
dominated and dependent. As it happens, he is presenting both forms as
'positive modes' of solicitude. He has already dealt with the 'deficient and
Indifferent modes' of solicitude, which occur especially when we are
'without one another, passing one another by, not "mattering" to one
another'. Even here he goes on to say that, if 'Dasein does *not* turn to
Others, and supposes that it has no need of them or manages to get along
without them, it *is* in the way of Being-with'. In existentialist terms, one
may be without others. In existential terms, one is never without others.

Heidegger is revealing his intent here. Once again it has to do with
Being. He is not expounding everyday meanings of solicitude but presenting
a phenomenology of Being-in-the-world. He is dealing with solicitude not
for its own sake as an action in the world but in order to explicate the
Being of *Dasein*. If there are 'deficient' and 'indifferent' modes of solicitude,
it is because they are imperfect forms of solicitude as 'a state of Dasein's
Being', not because they fail to measure up to some ethical standard.
Dasein means Being-there. It necessarily implies Being-in-the-world. But
Being-in, Heidegger says, 'is *Being-with* Others'. *Dasein*'s world is a 'with-
world'. It is in this context that he discusses solicitude and it leads him to
a discussion, not about being compassionate to others or empowering
others, but about being true to one's own self. What he relates solicitude
to is authenticity.

'Leaping ahead' gives back to others their potentiality for Being and so
'pertains essentially to authentic care'. It is part of a way of Being-with-one-
another whereby people 'become *authentically* bound together, and this
makes possible the right kind of objectivity, which frees the Other in his
freedom for himself'. Heidegger, we need to note, is speaking of freedom
for oneself. He is concerned with authenticity, which translates *Eigentlichkeit*
('one's very own selfness') and has to do with living to the full the truth of
one's own Being. Heidegger is simply describing our ways of being and
nowhere does he offer ethical prescriptions or advice. Even if Sartre is right
in saying that Heidegger's 'authentic' and 'inauthentic' 'are questionable
and not very sincere, owing to their implicit moral content',[45] and that

'such a classification is infected with an ethical concern by its very terminology, despite its author's intention',[46] this implicit content and this ethical concern do not relate to others but to ourselves. It does not have to do with being advocates for others or facilitators or empowerers of others. It has to do with being true to one's own being. As Kaelin puts it:

> Heidegger's excursion into our being with others ... is a step in his attempt to show that one may be concerned with the things of one's world in such a way as not to be oneself. Others are met in our worlds, as cited above, by what they do. They help us; they hinder us; or they are indifferent to our very existence.[47]

There is nothing, here or elsewhere, to warrant the claim of nurse researchers that Heideggerian phenomenology and hermeneutics have to do with discerning the meaning of everyday practices as if these are perceived to have value in themselves. More than that, the reference to authenticity (which for Heidegger, as has been said, has to do with living to the full the truth of one's own Being) challenges their further claim that the Heideggerian approach seeks to determine *shared* meanings and *common* practices.

Benner, to the contrary, is insistent that the focus be kept on these shared meanings and common practices. She reminds us that 'human beings always come to a situation with a story, a preunderstanding'. It is a background that is 'handed down and not individually derived'. It is for this reason that hermeneutics does not rest content with the unique and the singular but searches out what is common and shared.

> In fact, the meaning-giving subject is no longer the unit of analysis. Meaning resides not solely within the individual nor solely within the situation but is a transaction between the two so that the individual both constitutes and is constituted by the situation. Therefore, the unit of analysis is the transaction. This position, however, expects not only the unique or idiosyncratic but commonalities and recurring similarities and differences as well.[48]

Why this emphasis on what is common and shared? For one thing, Benner sees it as a rampart that will defend research against methodological individualism. Such individualism, she tells us, 'is avoided by finding commonality and therefore teleological explanation and prediction based on background skills, meanings, and practices shared in a people with a common history and common situations'.[49] More than that, this commonality is the background which 'gives individuals the conditions of their possibility and the conditions for their perceptions, for their actions, and so forth'. Where else is the researcher to start from?

> ... the researcher is a self-interpreting human being who participates in a shared background of common meanings that can be made public through dialogue (Heidegger, 1962; Palmer, 1969).[50]

Here, as elsewhere, Benner is citing Heidegger. Bringing together, as she does, the notions of background and pre-understanding, she not only attributes the idea of background pre-understanding to Heideggerian phenomenology but asserts that the 'full-blown notion of background preunderstanding is one of the major distinctions between Heideggerian phenomenology and Husserlian transcendental phenomenology'.[51] However, Benner's exposition of background preunderstanding is very hard to square with what we find in Heidegger's writings. Heidegger clearly uses the term 'pre-understanding' in a radically different sense and what he relates it to essentially is fore-structure, not background.

For a start, these two words are not synonymous. 'Background' and 'fore-structure' throw up very different conceptions of the possibilities they are said to ground. In Benner's view, it is background — 'handed down' meanings, skills and practices — that 'gives individuals the conditions of their possibility'. On this understanding, our possibilities stem from the past. They are due to the potentiality with which our cultural heritage, together with our personal experience within that heritage, has endowed us. Heidegger's conception is markedly different. Once we begin the phenomenological investigation of *Dasein*, human being emerges as primarily a projection towards possibilities and, as Heidegger sees it, our possibilities are a gift of the future, not the past. In Heidegger's 'existential analysis', Sadler points out, possibility is an existential term that contrasts with the notion of potentiality:

> Potentiality refers to something which is to emerge from the past, whereas possibility refers to the not-yet-being which might emerge; if it does, possibility will emerge out of the future.[52]

At the heart of this discordance is the fact that, for Heidegger, pre-understanding is a fore-structure, not a background. It consists, he tells us in his inimitable fashion, in a 'fore-having', a 'fore-sight' and a 'fore-conception'. Where Benner would search out common meanings as the starting point for her hermeneutics, Heidegger warns us that we must reach the fore-structure phenomenologically — by a return to 'the things themselves' — and not by accepting what happen to be the prevailing understandings.

> In the [hermeneutic] circle is hidden a positive possibility of the most primordial kind of knowing. To be sure, we genuinely take hold of this possibility only when, in our interpretation, we have understood that our first, last, and constant task is never to allow our fore-having, fore-sight, and fore-conception to be presented to us by fancies and popular conceptions, but rather to make the scientific theme secure by working out these fore-structures in terms of the things themselves.[53]

Heidegger's talk of 'fancies and popular conceptions' links to what he has to say a little later in *Being and Time* about idle talk.[54] Once again he insists that he is not being disparaging in referring to idle talk (or, if it is a matter of the written word, to scribbling). As always, his focus is ontological. Idle talk is talk that 'has lost its primary relationship-of-Being towards the entity talked about, or else has never achieved such a relationship'. For that reason, 'it does not communicate in such a way as to let this entity be appropriated in a primordial manner'. Instead of serving 'to keep Being-in-the-world open for us in an articulated understanding', idle talk serves 'to close it off, and cover up the entities within-the-world'. It interprets things for us and it does so in an authoritative way: 'Things are so because one says so.' It is the 'everyday way in which things have been interpreted' and it 'has already established itself in Dasein'.

Thus, Heidegger agrees with Benner that we bring shared meanings to any situation. There is a place in his exposition for a culturally derived 'background'. When he sets the stage for his analytic of Dasein, he does so against the backdrop of a shared world of meaning. He accepts that we start with 'average understanding', with 'the public way in which things have been interpreted'. Indeed, there is no other starting point.

> This everyday way in which things have been interpreted is one into which Dasein has grown in the first instance, with never a possibility of extrication. In it, out of it, and against it, all genuine understanding, interpreting, and communicating, all re-discovering and appropriating anew, are performed. In no case is a Dasein, untouched and unseduced by this way in which things have been interpreted, set before the open country of a 'world-in-itself' so that it just beholds what it encounters. The dominance of the public way in which things have been interpreted has already been decisive even for the possibilities of having a mood — that is, for the basic way in which Dasein lets the world 'matter' to it. The 'they' prescribes one's state-of-mind, and determines what and how one 'sees'.[55]

So the agreement with Benner, such as it is, is short-lived. As Heidegger's very language indicates, there is a profound difference in their respective accounts of the role and value of everyday meanings. For Benner, those everyday meanings are the target of hermeneutical endeavours. She sees them as founding our very possibilities. Heidegger, to the contrary, sees such everyday understanding as fancies and popular conceptions, the outcome of idle talk. The everyday understanding interprets for us. to be sure. However, far from opening us to Being, this 'interpretedness' closes Being off from us. Its only merit is that it offers us, from within its own depths, an authentic, albeit obscure and implicit, pre-understanding of Being.

> ... Dasein is constantly delivered over to this interpretedness, which controls and distributes the possibilities of average understanding and of the state-of-mind belonging to it. The way things have been expressed or spoken out is such that in the totality of contexts of signification

into which it has been articulated, it preserves an understanding of the disclosed world and therewith, equiprimordially, an understanding of the Dasein-with of Others and of one's own Being-in.[56]

The gap between Heidegger and Benner could hardly be wider, even if both of them use the same word, i.e. 'pre-understanding', to indicate their hermeneutical starting point. For Benner, as we have already noted more than once, this 'pre-understanding' is the 'background meanings, skills and practices'[57] one inherits. It is 'what a culture gives a person from birth ... a shared public understanding of what is'.[58] For Heidegger, the pre-understanding he talks of is a pre-understanding of Being. It is to be found, phenomenologically, in the shared public understanding where it is preserved, but otherwise this shared public understanding is to be seen as a seduction (no one is 'unseduced') and a dictatorship (we are subject to 'the dominance of the public way in which things have been interpreted'). This, Heidegger believes, is a dominance by *das Man*, i.e. the 'they', the anonymous 'One'. The interpretedness, the shared understanding, is not in itself the source of meaning and fulfilment that Benner makes it out to be. It is, instead, the *locus* where our dimly lit pre-understanding of Being may be divined and, for the sake of that pre-understanding and its explication, is to be left behind as, phenomenologically, we travel Heidegger's hermeneutic circle.

It will be helpful to explore Heidegger's thought about everydayness and *das Man* a little further. Let us look again at the hermeneutical task. As a pre-conceptual grasp of Being, the fore-structure forms the basis of a hermeneutical project that seeks to explicate the understanding of Being. What is shadowy and latent is to be brought into the clear light of day. This must be done phenomenologically. The return to the things themselves, Heidegger tells us, is 'our first, last, and constant task' and, for him, a return to the things themselves is a return to Being, for Being must always be 'the first and last thing-itself of thought'. Thus Kaelin writes of 'Heidegger's continual search for primordiality of ontological significance'.[59]

In other words, one must allow the structures of Being to present themselves. When that is done, the first insight gained is the understanding of *Dasein* as a projection towards possibilities, i.e. towards the future, thereby introducing the central and pervasive notion of temporality. This projection involves a comprehension of *Dasein* as Being-in-the-world, with the 'world' and 'care' as correlative phenomena. In the process various other existential structures come into view as the foundation of the possibilities to come. In the quotation given above, Heidegger is listing such existentials when he refers to 'world', 'Dasein-with' and 'Being-in'. Having elucidated the existential structures of our being, we can then return to our concrete existence in the world and discover our possibilities in the light of them.

Among the structures uncovered are 'averageness' and 'everydayness'. These are existentials that 'permit the human being to lose itself in a public world, acting conventionally as the impersonal self everyone must assume to adapt to such a world'.[60] Heidegger has much to say about this impersonal self. As already mentioned, he ascribes it to seduction and domination by *das Man*, the anonymous 'they' or 'One'. We come to live our lives guided and controlled by the social forces signified by *das Man*. This, for Heidegger, is inauthenticity.

> Dasein's everyday possibilities of Being are for the Others to dispose of as they please. These Others, moreover, are not *definite* others ... not this one, not that one, not oneself, not some people, and not the sum of them all. The 'who' is the neuter, *the 'they'* ...
>
> In this inconspicuousness and unascertainability, the real dictatorship of the 'they' is unfolded. We take pleasure and enjoy ourselves as *they* take pleasure, we read, see, and judge about literature and art as *they* see and judge; likewise we shrink back from the 'great mass' as *they* shrink back; we find 'shocking' what *they* find shocking. The 'they', which is nothing definite, and which all are, though not as the sum, prescribes the kind of Being of everydayness.[61]

Because the hermeneutic inquiry begins with human being in its averageness and everydayness, the self that first gets expressed is inauthentic in this sense. In viewing it in that light, Heidegger does not see himself as passing any moral judgment. He means simply that this self is not truly our own. What Heidegger looks for, then, is a way of uncovering *authentic* human being. Doing so turns out to be one aspect of the 'reversal' referred to earlier. We need to reverse the process. We have moved from consideration of *Dasein* to a description of the existentials. Now we must move from the existentials back to *Dasein* to discover authentic being as a possibility within our 'ontic', i.e. real-life, situation.

How Heidegger sees that being done is a complex account. It involves the possibility of 'resoluteness' as a way for a human being to be an authentic whole. This is an 'anticipatory' resoluteness, for it anticipates the ultimate possibility, death, which is for *Dasein* 'its ownmost possibility'[62] and beyond which there will be nothing. All possibilities are evaluated in the light of death as the supreme possibility: when one lives in the anticipation of death, one lives with a resoluteness which brings unity and wholeness to the self. Temporality is involved too — a move from the 'time of the world', which the inauthentic self embraces, to an original temporality that reflects the constancy of the authentic self called into existence by anticipatory resoluteness. It is in such resoluteness and constancy, and not in average everydayness, that Heidegger posits authentic human being.

There is profundity in Heidegger's thought here. It is not easy to come to terms with. Yet one thing is clear: invoking Heideggerian phenomenology or hermeneutics on behalf of a search for commonalities, as if such commonalities constitute the hermeneutical goal, is very much a distortion of what Heidegger is about.

Benner and the others do invoke Heideggerian phenomenology in precisely this fashion. Leonard, another nurse researcher, is a clear example.[63] She is one of many who expressly cite Benner in depicting Heideggerian hermeneutics as a search 'to find commonalities in meanings, skills, practices and embodied experiences'. Leonard states flatly, 'Private, idiosyncratic meanings are not the data of hermeneutic inquiry.' Leonard goes so far as to identify objectivity with sharedness and commonality.[64]

Why is Heidegger so routinely misconceived in nursing phenomenology? A clue to part of the answer can be found in Benner's statement, cited earlier, that Heideggerian phenomenology is 'a particular theoretical stance ... taken toward human beings and human experience'. Or in Watson's claim that one can derive from Heidegger's writings an 'existential phenomenological view of what it means to be a person'. Behind the dubious use of Heidegger in nursing phenomenology lies a certain concept of the person. It is a view of the person that nursing theorists unanimously espouse. It is attributed to Heidegger in these treatments of his hermeneutics but it bears little resemblance to the image of the human that emerges from his writings — or from his life.

Heidegger's image of the human

According to Patricia Benner,[65] Heideggerian phenomenology posits 'three essential tenets' relating to human beings.

First of all, human beings are 'self-interpreting' and their interpretations are 'constitutive of the self'.

Second, the kind of being that one is constitutes an issue for every human being. In short, we are each called to 'take a stand' on the kind of being we are.

Third, the self is not a radically free arbiter of meaning. While it is true that the meanings available to the individual can undergo transformation, they are limited by a particular language, culture, and history. Ours is a 'situated freedom and situated possibility'.[66]

It is interesting, and significant, that Benner chooses to describe human beings as self-interpreting rather than just interpreting. She is not alone is doing this. Taylor, whom she frequently cites, does the same, describing this as 'one of the basic ideas of Heidegger's philosophy, early and late'.[67] It may pass muster as a basic idea, but how primary it is in Heidegger's understanding of human being is another question. There is no doubt that, on the basis of Heidegger's writings, describing humans simply as 'interpreting beings' is much more faithful to his thought and emphasis. Heidegger's interest, as we have seen, is not primarily with any philosophical anthropology but with ontology in the most radical sense. Whatever the obscurities and complexities in the pages that follow, the Introduction to *Being and Time* states the aim of the treatise quite clearly: 'to work out the meaning of the question of *Being*'.[68]

So, if we want to add a prefix to the word 'interpreting', the word would have to be Being. In Heidegger, human beings are above all and before all Being-interpreters, seekers after the meaning of Being. In the 'Letter on humanism', *Dasein* is expressly presented as the 'shepherd of Being'[69] and the 'neighbour of Being'.[70] 'What counts', writes Heidegger, 'is *humanitas* in the service of the truth of Being.'[71] And, as Palmer points out in discussing Heidegger's *On the Way to Language*, 'thinking' (the word which came to the fore in Heidegger's later works as the word 'phenomenology' disappeared)[72] leads to Being rather than to the self.

> To put the matter in terms of expression and appearance, language is not an expression of man but an appearance of being. Thinking does not express man, it lets being happen as language event.[73]

While Heidegger is not given to describing human beings as 'self-interpreting', he does have something to say about 'self-knowledge' and a lot to say about 'self-understanding'. What one finds is that these terms link to knowledge and understanding of the world rather than to a focus on the self in itself and they look to future possibilities rather than to what the self might be here and now.

As far as Heidegger's use of 'self-understanding' is concerned, we should heed Hoy's warning[74] against positing some kind of Cartesian or Kantian ego at a remove from the objective world as if it occupied a different, subjective world. Hoy reminds us that, in Heidegger's view of things, world and *Dasein* are disclosed together, so that an understanding of the world is always also a self-understanding. Such self-understanding, then, is not a matter of discerning 'facts about the properties of a mental substance or a noumenal self'. It is a question of learning *Dasein*'s way of being in the world and dealing with the issue of its own existence. This is the point Heidegger makes when explaining his use of 'transparency' to designate self-knowledge:

> ... it is not a matter of perceptually tracking down and inspecting a point called the 'Self', but rather one of seizing upon the full disclosedness of Being-in-the-world *throughout all* the constitutive items which are essential to it, and doing so with understanding.[75]

Self-understanding, Heidegger also says, primarily relates to the future.[76] It stems from 'what can be' rather than from 'what is'.

Some caution is called for, therefore, in crediting Heidegger with the view that humans are self-interpreting beings whose interpretations are constitutive of the self. If it is legitimate at all to do so, the term 'self-interpretation' needs to be carefully nuanced.

Benner's second tenet holds that, in the philosophy of Heidegger, the kind of beings we are is presented to us as an issue and we are called to take a stand on that issue. This does seem, on the face of it, to make an existentialist of him, despite his protestations to the contrary. Many scholars are happy to do that. Indeed, it is not easy to read the early Heidegger in any other way. Even so, i.e. reading Heidegger in this way and taking the kind of beings we are to be a genuine 'issue' for us, we still need to ask what confronting this issue and taking a stand on it actually means. And that rather depends on how Benner's third tenet is understood.

For Benner, the issue is confronted in terms of our common heritage. It is there that we take our stand. That heritage may be limiting, but it also grounds our possibilities. There is for the individual, Benner assures us, no higher court than meanings or self-interpretations embedded in language, skills, and practices. There are no laws, structures or mechanisms that can offer higher explanatory principles or greater predictive power than the self-interpretations which we have in the form of common meanings, personal concerns and cultural practices shaped by a particular history.[77]

This is an optimistic account. 'People', says Benner, 'have direct access to meaningful situations by virtue of education and experience.'[78] To avail themselves of that access is to confront the issue of what kinds of being they are and to take a stand. Benner sees it as a rather straightforward process. She obviously wishes to keep it straightforward: there is to be no distraction from the description of 'lived meanings' by introducing alleged social or psychological (or, for that matter, ontological) factors.

> This is not a hermeneutics of suspicion, used by Marx or Freud or the mid-career Heidegger, where the goal is to discover some latent causal explanation in theoretical or power terms, such as class struggle, Oedipal complex, dependency needs, or anxiety over ungroundedness, but to accurately portray lived meanings in their own terms.[79]

While Benner dissociates herself from the 'mid-career Heidegger', it has to be said that the early and later Heidegger's account is not as straightforward as Benner's either — nor is it as optimistic. How does he suggest that we address the issue of what kind of beings we are? As we have seen already, it is by seeking authenticity, i.e. by being 'our own selves'. We take our stand by a choice of self. If that sounds straightforward enough, it should be kept in mind that, to be our own selves, we need an understanding of our identity. That, according to Heidegger, does not come easily. Authenticity is a notion Heidegger has taken from Kierkegaard and, referring to Kierkegaard's picture of authenticity, Solomon points out the greater pessimism and complexity to be found in Heidegger:

> Heidegger retains some of these features of authenticity, but he is by no means so sanguine as Kierkegaard about the identity of the individual. Making choices that are 'one's own' is far more problematic than it appears to be.[80]

As Heidegger sees it, we find ourselves 'thrown' into our world — abandoned in it, even. Despite this, we are able to make a choice of self. There are many things about which we have had no say but which stem, for instance, from heredity or society or history. For a start, we did not choose to be born. Nor did we choose our gender. And there are countless other factors which we have not chosen but which, as Heidegger puts it, are 'always already' there. Our existence in this 'always already' world he terms 'facticity'. Despite such facticity, we are not powerless. We may respond resolutely to the call of conscience and decide what we will do with the conditions established by our birth, our gender, and all the other unchosen circumstances. We can make a stand, taking over a range of possibilities that define our identity and constitute our future. When we do, Kaelin points out, Heidegger believes we are putting ourselves in charge of our situation and creating an authentic heritage for ourselves.

> Anticipating its end and retaining its past, not by remembering or forgetting, but by repeating the choice of itself, the resolute human being becomes master of its situation in the world ... It is in this way that it creates for itself a heritage, which it takes over in the constant repetition of itself — or rejects in losing itself within the public world.[81]

This heritage — our 'fate' — is the end result of a profound and demanding process. It has required, and continues to require, a resoluteness even 'towards death'. It means eschewing the control of *das Man*, a refusal to lose ourselves in a purely public world. Once achieved, this heritage overcomes the powerlessness we experience in being thrown into our world and forced to make choices among the possibilities we are offered. It is for us 'a moment of vision'[82] offering a perception of the structures of our personal existence.[83]

The possibilities coming to us out of the future, together with the resoluteness with which authentic individuals face them, constitute for Heidegger a self-understanding.

> In resoluteness the Dasein understands itself from its own most peculiar can-be. Understanding is primarily futural, for it comes toward itself from its chosen possibility of itself ... In resoluteness, that is, in self-understanding via its own most peculiar can-be — in this coming-toward-itself from its own most peculiar possibility, the Dasein comes back to that which it is ... [84]

Such self-understanding, as we have already noted, is a far cry from the 'interpretations' which Benner sees as 'constitutive of the self'. The kind of heritage she points to — the 'commonality and therefore teleological explanation and prediction based on background skills, meanings, and practices shared in a people with a common history and common situations'[85] — found for Heidegger only an inauthentic self and an inauthentic self-understanding. In that kind of self-understanding 'we are *not our own*, as we have lost our self in things and humans while we exist in the everyday'.[86]

Mind you, all this does sound mightily individualistic and daunting — an account of solitary individuals confronting their respective fates. According to Grene, the individual to whom Heidegger is pointing here is a 'rare man of character who has risen to the level of richer, more authentic existence, who has resolved in ruthless independence to fashion a life-toward-death, a freedom in finitude on his own pattern'.[87] Heidegger himself, Langan points out,[88] has described as 'extraordinary' the grasp of self required for authentic existence. At this point there is something very comforting about Benner's common culture and shared skills, practices and meanings.

Admittedly, Heidegger, in highlighting individuals' authentic existence, is not divorcing them from their fellows. Our actual situation is lived out under the ontological condition of our Being-with-others. Each of us may have a 'fate', but together we have a 'destiny'.

> ... if fateful Dasein, as Being-in-the-world, exists essentially in Being-with-Others, its historicizing is a co-historicizing and is determinative for it as *destiny*. This is how we designate the historicizing of the community, of a people. Destiny is not something that puts itself together out of individual fates, any more than Being-with-one-another can be conceived as the occurring together of several Subjects. Our fates have already been guided in advance, in our Being with one another in the same world and in our resoluteness for definite possibilities. Only in communicating and in struggling does the power of destiny become free. Dasein's fateful destiny in and with its 'generation' goes to make up the full authentic historicizing of Dasein.[89]

However, even with the emphasis Heidegger places on the destiny we share with our 'generation', the account remains a rather forbidding one and points up the sharp contrast to be found between the hermeneutics of Heidegger and the hermeneutics of Benner. By contrast, Benner's emerges as a highly humanistic account. A humanistic orientation, as understood in this context, is one characterised by a positive attitude towards human nature or human being. It gives pride of place to the human and does not hesitate to endow the human with intrinsic worth. Human being is valued for its own sake. From this viewpoint, there is a thoroughgoing humanism to be found in Benner. It is reflected in her view of humans as *self-interpreting* rather than as interpreters of Being. It is reflected in her locating possibilities in the person here and now rather than in what is to come. It is reflected in the whole context of communication, shared values and common meanings in which she sets her subjects. It is reflected in the optimism with which she views their task of attaining meaning and engaging in meaningful activity.

In the world which Benner addresses, people are free beings, albeit limited by their situation. They are equal beings, with inequality and the factors making for inequality expressly precluded as a 'hermeneutics of suspicion'. They are growthful beings too: in *The Primacy of Caring*, Benner and Wrubel begin their chapter 'On what it is to be a person' with a mini-case study in which, because nurse and nursing client learned to trust each other, the client learned to trust herself, and thereby 'the wholeness of her being emerged'.[90]

It is difficult to find humanism of this kind in Heidegger's philosophy. There one seems to be in a different world. Heidegger expressly denies that his project in *Being and Time* is humanistic, at least in the sense in which Sartre claims to be humanistic. Where Sartre is eager to brand his existentialism a humanistic philosophy (and a politically engaged humanism at that), Heidegger shows no such enthusiasm. Heidegger's 1946 'Letter on humanism' is addressed to his former student, Jean Beaufret, but is commonly considered to be provoked by Sartre's 'Existentialism is an humanism', if not a direct response to it. In this letter, Heidegger does not diverge from the image of the human he has been projecting up to this point. Each of us is called to dwell in the truth of Being. That is where true humanism lies, he asserts.

> 'Humanism' now means, in case we decide to retain the word, that the essence of man is essential for the truth of Being, specifically in such a way that the word does not pertain to man simply as such. So we are thinking a curious kind of 'humanism'.[91]

Heidegger is offering an understanding of authenticity and fulfilment that seems reserved for an élite. It summons up the vision of resolute, constant individuals who confront their thrownness and abandonment, responding to the stern call of conscience. Despite existential anxiety, they project themselves upon their possibilities. Thereby they reach their moment of vision and achieve their destiny in and with their similarly resolute and constant generation.

This is not the humanistic picture that the nursing phenomenologists paint. It would be surprising if it were. Heidegger, after all, was a Nazi. When he was elected Rector of the University of Freiburg in April 1933 (and at the same time appointed *Führer* of the University by the political authorities), he joined the Nazi party as of 1 May.

Heidegger made his inaugural address as Rector of the University on 27 May 1933. In this address Heidegger made repeated references to the 'fate' of the German people. It is the university which — 'from science and through science' — educates and disciplines the leaders and guardians of that fate. 'Science and German fate', he said, 'must come to power at *the same time* in the will to essence.' He went on to say that the 'much praised "academic freedom" is being banished from the German university;

for this freedom was false, because it was only negating'. In its place, the 'German student's notion of freedom is now being returned to its truth'. 'Out of this freedom', said Heidegger, 'will develop for German students certain bonds and forms of service.'[92]

This, some might say, was only the rhetoric expected from a University *Führer* on such an occasion. Can the same be said of Heidegger's letter to 'German students' published in a student newspaper six months later? In this letter he called upon students to display 'aggressive involvement in the struggle of the entire Volk itself' and concluded, 'The Führer alone *is* the present and future German reality and its law.'[93] It is hard to see this letter as anything other than Heidegger's own initiative. In fact, as Steiner observes, there was a spate of articles and speeches in 1933–34 in which Heidegger 'goes so crassly beyond official obligation, let alone a provisional endorsement'.[94] Caputo writes of 'his hellish endorsement of National Socialism and his ardent efforts to Nazify the German university'.[95]

At the end of the Second World War Heidegger was to portray his involvement with Nazism as a temporary liaison that quickly led to disillusionment and a severing of his ties with the party. He did resign as Rector on 23 April 1934. Some fourteen years later, well after the war had come to an end, Heidegger claimed that his resignation was 'in protest against the state and party'. He had acknowledged his political errors in 1934, he said, after expecting from National Socialism 'a spiritual rejuvenation of all life' and 'a rescue of Western existence from the danger of communism'.[96] He portrayed himself as an intellectual who had been under suspicion by the Nazi authorities and obstructed in publishing his writings.

On the basis of the available evidence (and it is evidence that has received a great deal of publicity in recent years, particularly through the work of authors like Farías and Ott),[97] it is difficult to dismiss Heidegger's involvement with National Socialism as merely a short-lived, albeit opportunistic, flirtation. Part of the evidence is the fact that Heidegger did not resign from the Nazi Party but remained a financial member until the end of the war. There is also the fact that, in a passage that he allowed to remain in the 1953 publication of *An Introduction to Metaphysics*, Heidegger, in referring to National Socialism, speaks of 'the inner truth and greatness of this movement'.[98] Even in the interview he gave to the German magazine *Der Spiegel* in 1966, to be published posthumously,[99] Heidegger offers no rejection of National Socialist principles. Indeed, while not at all sanguine that democracy can develop an adequate relationship with the essence of technology (a great preoccupation of Heidegger's), he credits National Socialism with some success in this regard.

Heidegger's resignation as Rector of the University followed strife with student bodies and argument over the deanship of the Law School. It was clearly not due to a rejection of National Socialism on his part. Four months after his resignation, we find him writing to Secretary of State Wilhelm Stuckart. Stuckart was attempting, unsuccessfully as it turned out, to develop an Academy of Professors of the German Reich. Heidegger wanted to become Director of this Academy. It was imperative, Heidegger's letter insisted, that the Academy's Director and its professors be not only National Socialist members but also 'National Socialist in spirit'.[100]

Heidegger's *An Introduction to Metaphysics* comprises the lecture series he presented in the summer semester of 1935. In these lectures National Socialism is said to be following the right path where Marxism and positivism had not. What had led National Socialism astray was not its racism but its espousal of inadequate principles. Here there is some indication that, while Heidegger was persisting in his support of National Socialism as such, there was a growing disillusionment on his part with the Nazi Party and the regime.[101] He was gravely disappointed with the way things had turned out for himself for he was totally thwarted in his political ambitions.

According to Farías, Heidegger's failure to realise his political aspirations stemmed from his identification with a discredited faction within the party. This faction, headed by Ernst Röhm and regarded as being to the Left, was in open opposition to the biological line of racism supported by Alfred Rosenberg and Ernst Krieck, who had the blessing of the party and enjoyed official standing within the bureaucracy. As Farías sees it, the revolutionary fervour of the Röhm faction proved to be a threat and the business interests supporting the party gave warning that the revolutionary moves of the Röhmists could no longer be tolerated. They were jeopardising alliances and plans still deemed to be necessary. This meant that Heidegger's support base was being eroded. A month or two after his resignation, Röhm was eliminated. The failure of the Röhm group put paid to Heidegger's political aspirations. After his resignation, he may well have been watched by the regime. If so, he would have been under scrutiny not as an opponent of National Socialism but as a representative of a factional element within it that had fallen into official disfavour.

By Heidegger's own account, he became convinced that the Nazis had become traitors to the truth that was at the root of their movement. Yet he continued to be regarded as a Nazi. In 1936, when he went to Rome (with government approval) to lecture at the Istituto Italiano di Studi Germanici, his former student at Marburg, Karl Löwith, was shocked to find him wearing Nazi Party insignia. 'At no time', writes Ott, 'did he adopt a position of protest.'[102]

Steiner underlines the fact that Heidegger never made a public recantation in regard to what the Nazi movement had done.[103] In this Steiner is echoing the sentiments of many people who are otherwise admirers of Heidegger's philosophy. It is known that the theologian Rudolf Bultmann (Heidegger's colleague in his Marburg days), the critical Marxist

Herbert Marcuse, and the existentialist Karl Jaspers all expressly urged him to make a public statement. The reasons why Heidegger failed to do so, says Krell, 'resist all explanation'.[104]

Krell tries his hand at explaining those reasons, nonetheless. He wonders, charitably, whether 'his reasons for refusing had more to do with a Kierkegaardian contempt for publicity and our media-dominated lives than with crass indifference'. Others would want to say that Heidegger failed to make such a statement because, to the very end, he remained a convinced and fervent National Socialist.

Farías writes:

> All those studies that attempt to minimize Heidegger's compromise with National Socialism or those wanting to see a deeper and more 'metaphysical' meaning in Heidegger show signs of a systematic unawareness of the texts where Heidegger speaks to us about his Nazi faith, tied to the person of Adolf Hitler.[105]

How closely linked, then, are Heidegger's philosophy and his politics? There seem to be intimate connections between Heidegger's frankly political Rector's Address in 1933 and the thought expressed in *Being and Time* six years earlier. In *Being and Time*, as we have seen, Heidegger points up the resoluteness demanded of individuals as they confront their personal fate now turned into communal destiny. This resoluteness is one that envisages death itself. It involves struggle and calls for an exemplary leader. For, when Heidegger tells us that the only authority for the free existing being is the 'repeatable possibilities of existence',[106] how is one to gauge what in the past is worthy of repetition? Not by remembering and assessing, but by choosing a hero who can endow past existence with an archetypal significance.[107] All this and much more in both *Being and Time* and his other writings prior to 1933 can be read as mirroring the Nazi rhetoric. Hans Ebeling insists that the notion of freedom in *Being and Time*, like that in National Socialism, leads to a radical denial of human equality,[108] while Steiner believes that in *Being and Time* the 'idiom of the purely ontological blends with that of the inhuman'.[109]

In the *Der Spiegel* interview of 1966, philosophy and politics are linked once more.[110] As we have seen, while admitting that the National Socialist movement was shackled by the philosophical ineptitude of its leaders, Heidegger continues to claim that National Socialism went some way towards addressing the problems posed by the uncontrolled mastery of technology (whereas he cannot say the same of democracy). And his German supremacism shines through. Not only does he suggest that the central problem of humanity must be solved in Europe ('where the modern technological world originated') but agrees that, in its solution, the Germans have a 'concrete destiny', a 'special task' and a 'special qualification'. Even the German language is an important instrument to this end. 'This has been confirmed for me today again by the French', Heidegger says. 'When they begin to think, they speak German.'[111]

The picture painted by writers like Farías, Steiner and Ott is not universally accepted by Heideggerian scholars.[112] Some accuse Farías of bias,[113] while Kaelin says that 'Steiner seems obsessed with Heidegger's "Nazism"'.[114] Much earlier Fell had written of 'a welter of slander' about Heidegger's Nazism.[115]

Others query the relevance of Heidegger's politics, content to divorce his philosophy from any questions about the morality of his political involvement. Richard Rorty, for example, while considering Heidegger to be 'a rather nasty piece of work', claims that 'there is no way to correlate moral virtue with philosophical importance or philosophical doctrine'. That we are talking about philosophy in particular makes no difference, as Rorty sees it. It does not matter that we are talking about an original philosopher rather than, say, an original mathematician or an original microbiologist or a consummate chess player. One must distinguish clearly between Heidegger's philosophical originality and importance, on the one hand, and deficiencies in Heidegger's moral character, on the other.[116]

Making a clear distinction of that kind is by no means easy. While Jacques Derrida is right in asserting that 'no one has ever been able to reduce Heidegger's thought in its entirety to that of a Nazi ideologue',[117] the extent to which one can treat Heidegger's political stance and his philosophy in isolation from one another is surely questionable. Guignol, for one, believes there is 'no way to buy into his philosophy without reflecting deeply on its moral and political implications', just as there is 'no way to make Heidegger's thought consonant with our own deepest democratic sentiments without distorting it'.[118] Sheehan echoes these sentiments: 'If Heidegger himself insisted that his engagement with Nazism came from the very essence of his philosophy', perhaps his followers should believe him..[119]

Heidegger certainly did so insist. When he met with Karl Löwith in Rome in 1936 and Löwith put it to him that his support of the Nazis emanated from the very essence of his philosophy, he agreed unreservedly. Löwith concludes:

> Given the significant attachment of the philosopher to the mood and intellectual habitus of National Socialism, it would be inappropriate to criticize or exonerate his political decision in isolation from the very principles of Heideggerian philosophy itself. It is not Heidegger, who, in opting for Hitler, 'misunderstood himself'; instead, those who cannot understand why he acted this way have failed to comprehend him.[120]

Heidegger's thought is abstruse, as we have seen. Even when we take due account of his life and actions, it is still very easy, in Löwith's term, to 'have failed to comprehend him'. Some things remain clear, nevertheless.

For one thing, Heidegger's life shows very clearly that one should not expect from him a warmly humanistic account such as is found in what the nursing literature presents as Heideggerian phenomenology or hermeneutics. He is not that kind of humanist and his phenomenology and hermeneutics are not that kind of enterprise. It is also clear that he cannot be invoked on behalf of a methodology that rests content with identifying shared meanings embedded in cultural practices and everyday narratives.

At the same time, who would deny that there is so much to learn from interacting creatively with Heidegger's thought? He is the most provocative of thinkers. Perhaps more than any other twentieth-century philosopher, he has succeeded in stimulating thought in others. We may eschew his form of humanism but engaging with it may well lead us to question the individualism, egocentricity and optimism of our own. We may find his fundamental ontology and even his 'history of being' inadequate reward for arduous efforts at 'phenomenological seeing'. Yet his phenomenology may at least encourage us to follow an authentic phenomenological path for our own purposes.

Our discussion began with some of the nursing phenomenologists considered in Chapter 1 who claim to be Heideggerian in approach. This discussion — circuitously, perhaps paradoxically — has set the scene for considering in broader terms the genesis of the new phenomenology which nursing research has embraced so wholeheartedly. If it is accepted that the new phenomenology does not coincide with mainstream phenomenology, including the hermeneutical phenomenology of Martin Heidegger, but is, in fact, radically different, the question at once arises: How has the new phenomenology come to emerge in the way it has? If it is not informed by phenomenological philosophy, what does inform it?

In attempting to answer such questions, we find the word 'humanism' continuing to intrude.

NOTES

1 'Phenomenology as defined by Martin Heidegger involves letting lived experience be revealed as it exists, without predetermined categories (Palmer, 1969). It affirms subjective experience, and is in contrast to the objectivity and reductionism sought through a positivist perspective. The nurse-researcher using this approach seeks to elucidate through dialogue turned into written text the clinical wisdom embedded in the everyday practice stories of nurses.' (Zerwekh 1992, p. 16)

2 'The existential phenomenological view of what it means to be a person presented in this study is derived primarily from the writings of Heidegger (1962), and also from the work of Benner and Wrubel (1989). Existential phenomenology does not seek to study individuals separately from the environment in which they live. To understand a person's experience, one

has to study the person in context, for it is only there that what a person values and finds significant is visible.' (Watson 1991, pp. 10–11)

3 'Heidegger extends phenomenology into the hermeneutical interpretation of the meaning of human experience in its situated context: cultural practices or shared meanings in which humans become humans form a contextual background against which and in which all human behaviour takes place. Hermeneutical inquiry is holistic in that the examination of any part of the phenomenon described is done while maintaining the context in which it occurs (Bleicher, Dreyfus).' (Dobbie 1991, p. 825)

4 '... a phenomenological approach to schooling in nursing. The approach is based on Heideggerian phenomenology ... It stems from researching the lived experience, a human science approach for research in phenomenological pedagogy ...'

'Heideggerian hermeneutics, first introduced to nursing by Benner, seeks to reveal the frequently taken for granted shared practices and common meanings embedded in our day-to-day lived experiences ...'

'Shared practices and common meanings were identified and coded as themes and constitutive patterns ... Since shared practices and common meanings are described, it is assumed they will be recognizable to the reader who shares the same culture ... Through understanding the lived experiences that reveal people's shared practices and common meanings, nursing education will be transformed.' (Diekelmann 1992, pp. 72–74)

5 'Heideggerian phenomenology seeks to make visible the nature and meaning of Being. Being is the being of whatever is; human being is just one manifestation of Being. We come to understand some of the possible meanings of Being through our experience of the world and our being within it. Everyday experience as it is lived is, thus, the focus of attention; the concern is to render lived experience intelligible as this is the place where meaning resides. Yet precisely because our lived experience is "everyday" and seems ordinary, much of its meaning remains hidden.'

'Heideggerian phenomenology holds that our foundational mode of existing as persons is in interpretation and understanding. Understanding is grasping one's own possibilities for being, within the context of the world in which one lives; understanding is a mode of being. Understanding is rendered explicit by interpretation, that is, in language. Language does not merely represent our way of being, it discloses what it is to "be". Language is a mode of human being which unveils Being. Hermeneutics means interpretation ... The goal of hermeneutical analysis is to discover meaning and achieve understanding ...'

'Hermeneutics means interpretation. Hermeneutics has been used since the early Greeks as a systematic approach to interpreting oral and written texts. However, Heidegger (1927/1962) stated that everyone exists hermeneutically, finding significance and meaning everywhere in the world. Heidegger saw that hermeneutic methods could, thus, be applied to our understanding of life and other persons, the everyday world of practices, and lived experience.' (Rather 1992, p. 48)

6 Pöggeler (1978), p. 97.

7 The word *Dasein* is a common German term, almost a colloquialism, for 'existence'. It means literally 'being-there'. Heidegger used it to denote human being, not as a human subject *per se*, but as the locus where Being manifests itself.

8 See Sartre (1956a).

9 Heidegger (1962), p. 32.

10 Boelen (1975), pp. 98–99. Edie (1964, p. xviii) makes much the same point: 'For Heidegger, on the contrary, it is not this world but the Being of beings which is the primary reality, and any analysis of human experience, perceptual or otherwise, is only a means to pose the more fundamental question of this Being.'

11 Heidegger (1962), p. 293.

12 *Ibid.*, p. 358.

13 *Ibid.*, p. 25.

14 *Ibid.*, p. 60.

15 *Ibid.*, p. 58.

16 *Ibid.*, p. 50.

17 In Richardson (1963), p. xiv.

18 See Boelen (1975), p. 100.

19 Heidegger (1971), pp. 10–11.

20 Heidegger (1962), pp. 61–62.

21 Richardson (1963), p. 631.

22 Diekelmann (1992), p. 73.

23 Benner (1985), p. 5.

24 *Ibid.*

25 Heidegger (1962), p. 50.

26 In Richardson (1963), p. xviii.

27 Heidegger (1962), p. 363.

28 *Ibid.*, p. 195.

29 Rather (1992), pp. 48–49.

30 Leonard (1989), p. 50.

31 Okrent (1988), p. 164.

32 Heidegger (1977c), p. 303.

33 Heidegger (1959), p. 14.

34 'Der Anfang -anfänglich begriffen — ist das Seyn selbst' (Heidegger 1989, p. 58).

35 Heidegger (1949c), p. 283.

36 *Ibid.*, p. 289.

37 *Ibid.*, p. 282.

38 Heidegger (1975), p. 12. Heidegger claims that the essence of poetry lies in thinking, but it is not easy to determine how he sees the relationship between poetry and thinking. As Luegenbiehl (1976, pp. 127–129) points out, 'Heidegger wants to assert that they can say the same only as long as a "chasm between poetry and thought gapes clearly and decidedly". (*Vorträge und Aufsätze* II, p. 12) Poetry and thinking live on the "most separate of mountains". (*Was ist das … die Philosophie*, 94) … Doing poetry is the task of poets. Thinking is the task of philosophers.' Heidegger's explanation of the paradoxical relationship between poetry and philosophy rests on an elucidation of 'sameness' as opposed to 'identity'.

39 After pointing out that the second half of *Sein und Zeit* had not yet appeared, Bochenski (1974, p. 164) observes, 'The *Brief über den "Humanismus"* and other new writings of Heidegger contains indications of a fundamental change in his thinking.'

40 Kaelin (1988), pp. 189–190, 192.

41 See Guignon (1993), pp. 6–7.

42 See Heidegger (1962), pp. 158–163.

43 See *ibid.*, p. 83.

44 Benner and Wrubel (1989), pp. 48–49.

45 Sartre (1956a), p. 531.

46 *Ibid.*, p. 564.
47 Kaelin (1988), p. 95.
48 Benner (1985), p. 7.
49 *Ibid.*
50 Benner (1984), p. 218.
51 Benner (1985), p. 6.
52 Sadler (1969), p. 75.
53 Heidegger (1962), p. 195.
54 *Ibid.*, pp. 211–214.
55 *Ibid.*, p. 213.
56 *Ibid.*, p. 211.
57 Benner (1985), p. 7.
58 Benner and Wrubel (1989), p. 46.
59 Kaelin (1988), p. 65.
60 *Ibid.*, p. 202.
61 Heidegger (1962), p. 164. Tiryakian dwells upon this theme: 'One does not care for what is original; originality is levelled down to familiarity. What is most profound and really secret loses its original distinction and becomes popularized or vulgarized; correlatively what is originally superficial is made profound — levelling is a two-way process. In this public world — this world of publicity — all is really unclear, ambiguous, hazy, yet everything is presented as if it were clear and well-known. We are afraid to ask questions which are not superficial for fear that One will think we are ignorant; in the realm of public life, ignorance is un-bliss. In the everyday world of the One, everything takes on a hue of soporific optimism. One always feels better, and things are always getting along well with One, things are always "fine".' (Tiryakian 1962, p. 128)
62 Heidegger (1962), p. 307.
63 See Leonard (1989).
64 *Ibid.*, p. 52.
65 Benner (1985), p. 5.
66 Benner and Wrubel (1989), p. 54.
67 See Taylor (1985), p. 45.
68 Heidegger (1962), p. 19.
69 Heidegger (1977b), pp. 210, 221.
70 *Ibid.*, p. 222.
71 *Ibid.*, p. 231.
72 See Spiegelberg (1982), p. 401.
73 Palmer (1969), p. 155.
74 Hoy (1993), p. 177.
75 Heidegger (1962), p. 187. Taylor too writes of this essential relatedness of subject to world, which Heidegger is emphasising here. As we have seen, Taylor considers that the notion of the human as a self-interpreting being remains central to Heidegger's thought. However, at least in a later work, his account reflects Heidegger's idea of 'self-understanding', i.e. with the focus not on 'a point called the Self' but on being-in-the-world. In discussing the making of the 'modern identity', Taylor talks of the shift to a 'new subjectivism' (a description he ascribes to Heidegger). This shift occurred with 'the modern idea of a subject as an independent existent ... it involves a new localization, whereby we place "within" the subject what was previously seen as existing, as it were, between knower/agent and world, linking them and making them inseparable' (Taylor 1989, p. 188).
76 Heidegger (1982), p. 287.

77 See Benner (1985), p. 5. Here Benner is using figurative language reminiscent of Merleau-Ponty; yet the two are poles apart. Their use of the same metaphor in such different ways points up rather strikingly the difference between the new phenomenology and mainstream phenomenology. For Benner, there is 'no higher court' than the meanings embedded in shared language, skills, and practices. On the other hand, Merleau-Ponty (1962, p. 23) states that the 'ultimate court of appeal' in our knowledge of things is our *experience* of them (and he makes it clear that he is speaking of our immediate experience, i.e. the 'phenomenal field' or what he has earlier described as 'direct and primitive contact with the world').

78 Benner (1985), p. 8.

79 *Ibid.*, p. 6.

80 Solomon (1988), p. 161.

81 Kaelin (1988), p. 238.

82 Heidegger (1962), pp. 376, 387, 437, 442.

83 See Kaelin (1988), pp. 237–239.

84 Heidegger (1982), p. 287.

85 Benner (1985), p. 7.

86 Heidegger (1982), p. 160.

87 Grene (1960), p. 70.

88 See Langan (1966), p. 34. Langan goes on to describe what this grasp of self means for Heidegger. 'The true Self, the caring Self, the Dasein who understands himself in the structural whole of his Being as temporality, realizes itself as conscience (*Gewissheit*). Conscience suggests a note of awareness, the kind of awareness that is born of a steady gaze directed at things as they are. The German *Gewissheit* translates this note better, for the stem *Gewiss* basically signifies certitude. What is the nature of this certitude that opens the Dasein into the authentic existence of a life of conscience? It is the certitude of death as it is known by the *Sein-zum-Tode*. Conscience understood thus fundamentally is not a voice calling from outside, but a still and resolute address of the authentic Dasein to himself. This call (*Ruf*) is the voice of care (*Sorge*). It is call to salvation from the daily self-loss in 'what *they* say' ... Two notions, guilt and resolution, grow so intimately out of the one integral analysis of the Self that it is difficult to explain the one without the other. (*Ibid.*, pp. 35–37)

89 Heidegger (1962), p. 436.

90 Benner and Wrubel (1989), p. 27.

91 Heidegger (1977b), pp. 224–225.

92 See Heidegger (1991a).

93 See Heidegger (1991b).

94 Steiner (1978), pp. 116–117.

95 Caputo (1993), pp. 276–277.

96 In Farías (1989), p. 284.

97 See Farías (1989) and Ott (1993).

98 Heidegger (1959), p. 199.

99 See Heidegger (1991c).

100 In Farías (1989), pp. 199.

101 The disenchantment may have come somewhat later than this lecture series of 1935, all the same. There is some evidence that, despite denials that he had done so, Heidegger added words to this passage in *An Introduction to Metaphysics* when it was published in 1954. These words, given in parenthesis, have been read as toning down the provocative reference to 'the inner truth and greatness' of National Socialism. It has been suggested that, by doing so,

'Heidegger disingenuously misrepresented his later *critical* interpretation of National Socialism (one that would emerge from his Nietzsche lectures of the late 1930s) as a view he already held in 1935'. See the Introduction to Habermas (1991).

102 Ott (1993), p. 292.

103 '... nauseating as they are, Heidegger's gestures and pronouncements during 1933–4 are tractable. It is his complete silence after 1945 on Hitlerism and the holocaust which is very nearly intolerable.' (Steiner 1978, pp. 116–117*)*.

104 Krell (1989), p. 130.

105 Farías (1989), p. 117.

106 Heidegger (1962), p. 443.

107 See *ibid.*, p. 437. This is discussed in Harries (1978), p. 311.

108 'The egocentric solipsism that recognizes only the *in*equality of peoples, not their equality, was entrenched in 1927 in as total a way as it was in 1933. There is in *Being and Time* a kinship with ruthless anarchy just as there is in Heidegger's Rector's Address a kinship with the totalitarian state. In both cases the power of acknowledging the other as the other, as essentially equal, is missing, and for that reason it only remains to oppress the other without any leniency.' (H Ebeling, in *Freiheit, Gleichheit, Sterblichkeit.* Cited in Farías (1989), p. 62.)

109 Steiner (1978), p. 118.

110 See Heidegger (1991c).

111 This German supremacism was nothing new. Twenty-three years earlier, for example, in the 1943 summer lecture course on Heraclitus, Heidegger had this to say: 'The planet is in flames. The essence of humanity is out of joint. World historical reflection can only come from the Germans, assuming that they find and preserve 'what is German'. That is not arrogance, rather it is the knowledge of the necessary arrangement of an originary need.' (Cited in Pöggeler 1991, p. 206)

112 See Lavine (1990), Hindess (1992).

113 See Wolin (1991), pp. 286–290. In particular, Wolin criticises Farías' characterisation of Heidegger as not only a Nazi but a *radical* Nazi, i.e. an adherent of the Röhm faction. Wolin believes that this contention is 'far from persuasive' and that 'Farías has failed to provide adequate proof' (p.288).

114 Kaelin (1988), p. 338.

115 Fell (1979), p. 441.

116 See Rorty (1988).

117 Derrida (1991), p. 266.

118 Guignon (1993), p. 36.

119 Sheehan (1993), p. 92.

120 Löwith (1991), p. 182. Bernstein (1991) believes that the published memoirs and recollections of Löwith, along with those of Jaspers and the studies of Farías, Ott and Pöggeler, give us 'a more detailed and accurate account of what Heidegger said and did, as well as an increased awareness of his evasions, misleading statements, and crucial silences' (p.80). On the question of Heidegger's silence about Nazi atrocities, Bernstein claims that, once we grasp the hidden logic of his thinking, we become very aware that, in fact, he is *not* silent — or, rather, that his silence becomes 'resounding, deafening and damning' (pp.134–136).

5

Phenomenology and humanism

Readers who turn from studies in applied phenomenology to nursing phenomenology find themselves in a different world. Compare the two and there is little doubt that mainstream phenomenologists and nursing phenomenologists are engaged on different tasks.

For a start, nursing phenomenologists are clearly researching human subjects, not just human 'topics' or 'issues'. Their interest lies first and foremost with a particular group of people and those counterparts for whom the findings will have relevance. It is in terms of these specific persons that the research is being carried out.

Mainstream phenomenologists, to the contrary, are engaged with a phenomenon rather than with a particular person or group of people. They may well believe, with great passion even, that in the end their phenomenological endeavours will be of great benefit to people. After all, they are elucidating human phenomena, i.e. phenomena which living, breathing human beings encounter, must make sense of, and have to come to terms with. Here and now, however, any involvement with a particular group of people is for the sake of illumining the phenomenon, not the other way round.

Applied phenomenology

Take Max Scheler (1874–1928) for example. Scheler was a member of both the Munich and the Göttingen Phenomenological Circles that developed around Husserl in the first decade of this century. Scheler's primary interest was in philosophical anthropology, but he ventured as well into sociology and psychology. Where Husserl thinks of Being within the framework of logic and Heidegger conceives of Being in transcendental terms as beyond categorisation, Scheler considers Being in the context of persons. For this reason, he sets the highest premium on concrete personal experience and it is not surprising that he grasps phenomenology as the tool he needs to elaborate his understanding of what it means to be human. Like other phenomenologists, he looks to the self-givenness of phenomena, but he does not believe that what gives itself to us in immediate experience comprises essences divorced from life. Instead, he writes of 'value essence' (*Wertwesen*), seeing values as constituting the essences of things and seeking phenomenological intuition into precisely such essential values.[1] For Scheler, values and feelings are revelatory and they are explored in his thought to an extent not matched among his phenomenological contemporaries.

The outcome of this emphasis is a number of essays dealing with phenomena like sympathy, humility, resentment, repentance and shame. Scheler's study of shame[2] is of particular interest, since shame is a phenomenon that engaged the interest of several other German philosophers, including Nietzsche and Schopenhauer.

It is not difficult for us to summon up the picture of a piece of phenomenological nursing research focusing on shame. 'The lived experience of shame: a phenomenological study', it might well be headed. Such a study would centre on a specific group of subjects, perhaps hospitalised nursing clients who are required to undergo a particularly embarrassing medical or nursing procedure. These subjects would be asked to describe a situation in which they felt ashamed. They would be invited to express all their feelings, thoughts and attitudes. The common themes in their descriptions would be sought out and perhaps articulated in an 'exhaustive description', a 'general-level description', or a 'constitutive pattern'. Throughout the study this particular group of subjects being researched would remain central. The researcher would make every effort not to impose meanings or constructions on what these people have to say. And there may well be a disclaimer somewhere in the paper, pointing out that this is qualitative research and the findings, unlike those claimed for quantitative research, are not to be taken as generalisable. In short, they are findings about *this* group of people in relation to *their* experience of shame.

Scheler's phenomenological study of shame is nothing like that. Not once does he refer to people with whom he has worked in order to gain the understanding of shame he is presenting. This is not to say that he has worked it out alone. He has not played the part of the 'solitary, individual philosophiser' that Husserl spoke about. Scheler was not like Husserl in this respect. Where Husserl tended to work alone and even his daily walks with others, ostensibly for dialogue, turned out to be a series of monologues, Scheler was gregarious and interactive. Early on he used the Phenomenological Circles as his sounding board, but his milieu of preference was the café society of his day. There he would engage in warm and fruitful discussion with his peers and his followers. Scheler may not have 'done' research as we know it. In his phenomenologising there were no research committees or ethics boards! Still we can assume that his phenomenology of shame, like other examples of his applied phenomenology, was tried out on numerous human subjects — or, rather, tried out *with* and *by* numerous human subjects, for each would be doing a phenomenology. But there is no mention of this in Scheler's account of shame. It is not pertinent. He has not set out to describe these people. What he is describing is the phenomenon of shame, i.e. shame as it appears in immediate, primordial awareness out of a direct, intuitive relationship with it. 'In the phenomenological attitude', he tells us, 'what is meant is intuited. It is not observed.'[3] And the phenomenon he discovers is a human phenomenon. It is not presented as something peculiar to a specific group of people.

Beginning his phenomenological inquiry (which Emad has elucidated for us in close detail and describes as an 'excellent example of applied phenomenology'),[4] Scheler finds shame associated with other human feelings that turn us back on ourselves and enable us to feel our own selves. There is a sense of 'protectiveness of the self' about these feelings, including shame. Furthermore, shame seems to share with pride an awareness of one's own value and with humility the tendency towards devotion and loyalty. It is also very close to both repentance and the feeling of honour. There are dynamics to be perceived here, a dialectic. Scheler finds that shame embodies the tension of higher and lower levels of consciousness.

These preliminary notions come to the fore when Scheler more directly approaches the task of delineating the essence of shame. Because it appears as a turning-back-to-the-self in the tension of higher versus lower levels of consciousness, Scheler sees shame appearing in two modes: as a spiritual feeling of shame, and as a bodily shame. The one cannot be reduced to the other. While Scheler is led by these phenomenological insights to reject the eighteenth-century theory that attributes the genesis of shame to training and education, he sees that its 'expressional forms' are determined by tradition.

There is an unreflective association of shame with sex and this leads Scheler to devote considerable effort to clarifying the relationship. Scheler's phenomenological scrutiny of shame reveals that it has priority over the sexual drive and is not reducible to it. On the basis of this insight, Scheler does battle with Freud.

While this is to touch very skimpily on what is a profound treatment of the phenomenon of shame, enough may have been said to indicate the difference between Scheler's study of shame and the kind of research that nursing phenomenologists would tend to carry out on 'the lived experience of shame'. The reasons why nursing phenomenologists engage in research have to do, typically, with the nurses they represent or the clients they serve. They would study shame in order to know their clients or themselves better. It would undoubtedly be helpful for nurses to know why and how their clients experience shame, or why and how they themselves experience shame. In short, they do their research for very clear reasons external to the phenomenon involved. Given such purposes, the researchers are unlikely to perceive any need for a direct study of the phenomenon as such. Emad makes it clear that Scheler's *modus procedendi* is very different:

> Scheler, on the contrary, is not concerned with shame for this or that reason. His motive in studying shame is to disclose its *essential structure* and hence to work out its phenomenological foundation.[5]

This is not to say that Scheler recognises no usefulness in his work. He is concerned throughout to develop a philosophical anthropology that will assist us to understand what it means to be human. And he is interested in human values to a degree that may well be unparalleled among other phenomenologists. For all that, his study remains an objective study of shame, albeit sought within the subjective experience of shame. Because it is set within subjective experience and derives from it, such a study is not objective in the sense in which some scientists still claim their work to be objective, but it does not rest in the mere subjectivism of immediate individual feeling either. Asher Moore pinpoints this distinction:

> Nor must we forget that it is not the feeling or volition or action which is the illumination, but the reflective recapturing of it. We lose the phenomenon if, like a certain bad sort of science, we treat feelings as merely objects. But on the other hand, as long as we remain incarnated in their pure immediacy, we never achieve any phenomenon to lose.[6]

In Moore's terms, it can be said that, in dealing with feelings, the new phenomenologists 'remain incarnated in their pure immediacy'. Not so Max Scheler or the phenomenological movement generally. Scheler's treatment of shame is an attempt at a 'reflective recapturing of it'.

It is perhaps safe to say that not too many nursing phenomenologists would feel completely at home with Scheler's study of shame. The same could be said of Heron's 'phenomenology of social encounter: the gaze'.[7] Heron sees eye contact, the meeting of someone's gaze, as a significant aspect of social encounter. It is 'simultaneous reciprocal interaction' in a way that speaking and listening cannot be, since 'conversation between two persons is necessarily a serial exchange of speech', with speaking and listening more or less alternating. Proceeding in phenomenological fashion, Heron explores 'moments when gaze meets gaze'. He finds three features of the gaze one thus meets:

- its luminosity or 'gaze-light' in which the other person reveals his or her presence to me

- its 'streaming' quality whereby it seems to enter me and fill me out (thus Martin Buber wrote of 'the streaming human glance in the total reality of its power to enter into relation')[8]
- its meaning, for 'the gaze can be the bearer of a wide range of meanings'.

Heron links these three features to three ways in which one can direct consciousness. These ways have themselves been arrived at phenomenologically, i.e. they are derived from the experience of directing one's own gaze as a form of 'attending'. The three ways are:

1 directing awareness *from one area of experience to another*, e.g. from perception to memory, or from fantasy to reflective thinking
2 directing awareness *to an object within a distinct area of experience*, e.g. to this tree within one's field of vision, or to a deity within the sphere of worship, or to such-and-such a problem within the sphere of reflective thinking
3 directing awareness *in a particular mode* to an object within an area of experience, e.g. to a deity reverentially or sceptically, or to a memory descriptively or evaluatively.

Heron sees what he is doing as

> **... a radically constituted empiricism, in which the whole man** as both intellectual and sensitive being seeks to find the basic phenomenal categories which do justice to his most intensely lived experiences and seeks also to specify the conditions under which experiences occur.[9]

Would it be too much to say that, by and large, nursing phenomenologists could read Scheler's phenomenology of shame, Heron's phenomenology of the gaze, or other mainstream phenomenological studies, and perceive little or no affinity to what they themselves do? If that is the case, let us consider another account, one that they would undoubtedly relate to since it coincides in essential fashion with what they are about. It is an account of empathy.

The role of humanistic psychology

> Can I let myself enter fully into the world of his feelings and personal meanings and see these as he does? Can I step into his private world so completely that I lose all desire to evaluate or judge it? Can I enter it so sensitively that I can move about in it freely, without trampling on meanings which are precious to him? Can I sense it so accurately that I can catch not only the meanings of his experience which are obvious to him, but those meanings which are only implicit, which he sees only dimly or as confusion?

One can readily imagine the nurse researchers from Chapter 1 putting these precise questions to themselves as they prepare to carry out their interviewing. This series of questions sums up very well the purpose of their research as they articulate it and, in the light of that purpose, the need they perceive to obtain a 'first-person description', see things from the respondent's 'frame of reference', and thus capture (or perhaps uncover, for it may be implicit or vague) the meaning of the respondent's 'subjective experience'.

The passage that has been quoted here does not come from the pen of a nursing phenomenologist. They are the words of Carl Rogers,[10] who played such a crucial role, along with Abraham Maslow, in the emergence of humanistic psychology in the United States. Rogers is referring to his understanding of empathy, a concept which remains central to his psychotherapy as he moves from his non-directive approach, through a client-centred phase in the development of his thought and practice, to his final person-centred orientation.

According to Rogers, when I have empathy or 'empathic under-standing', I am 'sensing the feelings and personal meanings which the client is experiencing in each moment' and 'can perceive these from "inside", as they seem to the client'.[11] What I must try to do, though Rogers admits it is no easy achievement, is 'to understand an individual, to enter thoroughly and completely and empathically into his frame of reference'.[12] Here I need a relationship with the client that is characterised by 'a deep empathic understanding which enables me to see his private world through his eyes'.[13]

The correspondence between Rogers' view of empathic understanding and what nursing phenomenologists are doing is undeniable. Some actually use the word 'empathy' when describing how they go about their data collection. Dobbie's account, for instance, is undiluted Rogerian interviewing, and the early Rogers at that.

> Empathy was conveyed by attending to each woman through main-taining eye contact, an open face on posture and responding to verbal narratives with frequent 'um hums'. Reflective silences and repetition of statements often prompted continuing exploration by the women.[14]

That nursing phenomenologists should link Rogers' notion of empathy to phenomenology as they understand it is not surprising. Rogers himself makes this link. When describing the three kinds of knowledge his theory postulates,[15] he distinguishes 'subjective' knowledge (a way of knowing that relates to our own inner states), 'objective' knowledge, (a way of knowing that relates to the outside world) and a way of knowing that has to do with other people's inner states. What validates this third form of knowledge is empathic understanding, for it enables us to enter into other people's private world of meanings. Significantly, Rogers calls it 'interpersonal' or 'phenomenological' knowledge.

Underpinning Rogers' pivotal notion of empathy and the therapeutic approach it informs is a particular view of human being and inter-subjectivity. This, it can be argued, is very much the understanding embodied in phenomenological nursing research. To support this argument, we might consider the six principles which Arnett and Nakagawa[16] have identified in Rogers' concept of 'empathic listening'. According to these authors, the same six principles are to be found throughout the literature of humanistic psychology generally. What about nursing phenomenology, then? Are the six principles to be found there also?

The first of these principles is 'a normative emphasis on a subject's *unmediated, personal and direct experience* of others' internal states'. The normativeness, Arnett and Nakagawa point out, transcends social constraints such as facades, roles, conventions or artifices. This is undoubtedly reflected in nursing phenomenology. Not once in the thirty pieces of research examined in Chapter 1 is any doubt raised about the ability of the researcher to experience, via direct communication, the internal states — the 'perceptions, feeling and attitudes' — of the subjects of the research. Nor was any doubt ever raised about the openness, veracity, or depth of self-understanding of the subjects.[17]

Secondly, Arnett and Nakagawa talk of the 'concomitant concern for accurately reflecting the internal experience of oneself *and* the other'. In Chapter 1 we noted at some length the concern on the part of nursing phenomenologists — an overriding concern, in fact — to portray the experiences described by the subjects as accurately as possible. Rogers' preoccupation with reflecting one's own internal experience springs from the therapeutic character of the relationship. For a successful counselling relationship, he was fond of saying, one must be 'real'.

Thirdly, there is the 'assumption of the innate goodness of the human being'. The attitude of the Rogerian counsellor is one of 'unconditional positive regard' for the client. Inherent in this is a view of the person as an essentially growthful being. Indeed, the belief that every human being possesses an innate tendency towards self-realisation or self-actualisation has come to be the hallmark of humanistic psychologists, at least as the textbooks see them.

Nursing phenomenology too, and nursing itself as a profession and a discipline, tends to have a very positive view of human being and human fulfilment. If the roadblocks can be removed, growth and fulfilment will surely follow. Mention has already been made of Benner and Wrubel's introductory mini-case study about a nursing client for whom 'the wholeness of her being' was able to emerge. This outcome is attributed to the development of mutual trust between client and nurse, which in turn enabled the client to trust herself. Such a case study mirrors rather precisely the kind of accounts frequently found in Rogers and other humanistic psychologists.

The fourth principle that Arnett and Nakagawa highlight is that of 'presentness'. One must be present to the other. This is a call, they say, to '*active* participation, involving openness, risk-taking, disclosure, and receptivity'. This emphasis too is to be found in nursing phenomenology. It is reflected in another mini-case study used by Benner and Wrubel. This is a nurse's account of how she related to Lara, a cancer patient undergoing chemotherapy, and it opens Benner and Wrubel's chapter on 'A phenomenological view of stress and coping'. In this case study the nurse states her conviction that 'Lara was able to open up to me because I shared a piece of myself'. She tells of giving Lara 'unspoken permission to be angry or depressed; to question ... ' 'I was always open with her,' she says, 'accepted her feelings, and never made light of them.'[18] Those familiar with the thrust of humanistic psychology will recognise this nurse's approach at once. That this account should head a chapter dealing with a 'phenomenological view' is significant.

The emphasis on 'presentness' is reflected also in what some of the researchers considered in Chapter 1 have to say. 'The researcher', says Rose,[19] 'makes contact with the verbalized experiences of the participant only when listening with her total being and entirety of personality.' Dobbie is citing Massarik when she states that the phenomenological interview

> ... is characterized by maximal mutuality of trust, attaining a genuine and deeply experienced caring between interviewer and interviewee, and a commitment to joint research for shared understanding.[20]

Fifthly, Arnett and Nakagawa talk of '*equality* of participants' experience, with avoidance of power, coercion, and manipulation'. This too is stressed in nursing phenomenology. Dobbie refers to her respondents as 'co-researchers'. 'The dialogue', says Rose, 'is between two persons of equal level without social or professional division.'[21] And Wood, citing Rosenbaum's citation of Leininger (nurse researchers, both of them), insists:

> The researcher using a qualitative approach does not attempt to control or manipulate the individuals of interest to the study.[22]

Finally, according to Arnett and Nakagawa, a '*non-evaluative*, supportive climate' is called for. The listener is to withhold value judgments and demonstrate a capacity to listen without anticipating, interfering, competing, refuting, or warping meanings into preconceived interpretations. Observance of this principle is inherent in the nursing phenomenologists' use of 'non-directive', 'open-ended' and 'unstructured' interview methods and their earnest efforts to 'bracket' their presuppositions and preconceptions.

Thus, there is a striking concordance here between humanistic psychology, on the one hand, and the new phenomenology, embraced so wholeheartedly by nurse researchers, on the other. This concordance forms the basis of the claim being made here: that humanistic psychology has played a very significant role in determining how phenomenology has been understood and phenomenological research undertaken in North America and, following its lead, in the English-speaking world generally.

Humanistic psychology emerged as an organised movement in the United States in the early 1960s. Its roots go back much earlier. Around the turn of the century William James was deploring the atomism that had emerged in psychology. James looked for a scientific psychology that would preserve the wholeness of persons. Some decades later Gordon Allport propounded a thoroughgoing humanism in his approach to personality. Then the 1940s and 1950s saw psychologists like Abraham Maslow and Carl Rogers sharing a positive view of persons and interpersonal relationships. For them, the paramount task of psychology is to promote growth and development towards the realisation of human potentiality and the achievement of human fulfilment.

At that time psychoanalysis remained dominant in the realm of psychotherapy, although the movement by some away from Freudian orthodoxy and rewarding developments in ego psychology deserve to be noted. Within the universities and other laboratories it was the behaviourist model that reigned supreme. There psychologists were busily experimenting on rats and other animals, even the human variety. Viewing these two alternatives in contemporary psychology, some professionals (Rogers and Maslow were among them) felt the need for a 'Third Force' in psychology. Thus was born the movement that came to be known as humanistic psychology.

Its birth was presaged by a landmark call to reform by Maslow in 1957. He demanded that psychology be more concerned with the problems of humanity and less with the problems of 'the Guild'. The discipline's concern to be seen as 'scientific' had led, he felt, to its domination by questions of means and methods, so that it focused, not on what is important to persons and society, but on what appears amenable to a scientific mode of inquiry. Psychology must become more positive, bolder, more creative, he said. And, in a clear allusion to the behaviourist approach from which he had sprung, Maslow called on psychology to study the depths of human nature and not rest content with examining surface behaviour.[23]

Following this call to arms, a group of like-minded psychologists launched the *Journal of Humanistic Psychology* in 1961 and the following year saw the first conference of the American Association for Humanistic Psychology. The Association's Charter expressed the meaning that the 'humanism' of its title held for it:

- A centering of attention on the experiencing *person* and thus a focus on experience as the primary phenomenon in the study of man. Both theoretical explanations and overt behavior are considered secondary to experience itself and to its meaning to the person.

- An emphasis on such distinctively human qualities as choice, creativity, valuation, and self-realization, as opposed to thinking about human beings in mechanistic and reductionist terms.

- An allegiance to meaningfulness in the selection of problems for study and of research procedures, and an opposition to a primary emphasis on objectivity at the expense of significance.

- An ultimate concern with and valuing of the dignity and worth of man and an interest in the development of the potential inherent in every person. Central in this view is the person as he discovers his own being and relates to other persons and to social groups.[24]

Phenomenological psychology

Although the word 'American' was soon dropped from the title of the Association, humanistic psychology was, and has remained, very much a North American phenomenon, even if it has radiated to other Anglophone countries. In continental Europe, long before humanistic psychology emerged on the other side of the Atlantic, humanism in psychology had taken the form of phenomenological psychology.

This phenomenological psychology represents the confluence of a number of streams.

Some of the streams emanate from Brentano rather than Husserl. Carl Stumpf stands at the headwaters of one such stream. Stumpf, a student of Brentano at Vienna and a teacher of Husserl at Halle, understood phenomenology after his own fashion. All the same, he played a decisive role in the introduction of phenomenology into psychology and thereby had a particular impact on the Gestaltists. Experimental phenomenology is regarded as beginning with Stumpf. Another non-Husserlian current originates with the Graz School, the first psychological laboratory to be established in Austria. The Graz School was founded in 1894 by Alexius Meinong, another of Brentano's students. Meinong's views diverged from those of Brentano and he followed this up with some earnest feuding with Husserl. Because of this, the Graz School developed along independent lines, though in many respects it paralleled the course taken by the phenomenological psychology which developed out of the more central phenomenological movement stemming from Husserl.

Husserl's direct influence on psychology began at Göttingen where students of psychology came into contact with his ideas. Among these were Ernst Jaensch and especially David Katz who, Spiegelberg points out,[25] developed phenomenological psychology in a highly original way. Katz's phenomenology led him to a profound exploration of colour and touch. In each case it revealed a distinction between 'film' phenomena, which do not relate to three-dimensional space, and 'surface' phenomena, which do. Katz's phenomenological inquiry was particularly fruitful in the area of touch, which he saw as having more cognitive value than sight or hearing. For him, touch data are not only extraordinarily diverse but constitute for the subject an organised 'world' of experience. He also pointed to a class of touch data that are 'transparent' in that we can touch *through* them. Already the difference between this kind of approach in psychology and that adopted by humanistic psychologists should be coming to the fore.

Albert Michotte is another psychologist who is significant in the history of phenomenological psychology. Michotte, a Belgian, is associated chiefly with the University of Louvain. However, it was while working at Oswald Külpe's centre at Würzburg during 1907–08 that he came into contact with the ideas of Brentano, Meinong, Stumpf and others. His subsequent work at Louvain reflects this influence. Michotte did not involve himself directly with phenomenological philosophy. This is somewhat ironic, given that it was at Louvain that the Husserlian archives were established in 1939 after the Franciscan, Fr H L van Breda, succeeded in smuggling Husserl's papers out of Nazi Germany to save them from destruction as the work of a non-Aryan. Michotte used experimental techniques to explore the phenomena experienced by his subjects as thoroughly as possible and in all their concreteness. Working in this fashion, he studied such phenomena as causality, materiality and permanence.

After the Second World War, phenomenological psychology continued unabated in continental Europe with psychologists like Metzger in Germany, Buytendijk and Strasser in The Netherlands, and Kunz and Keller in Switzerland.

On the psychiatric side, phenomenology already had a long history. Mention has been made of Karl Jaspers' use of phenomenology in his psychopathology. Jaspers, referred to by Spiegelberg as 'the Brentano of phenomenological psychopathology',[26] drew on Husserl's *Logical Investigations*. He also sent Husserl copies of some of his studies and met with him in 1913 and 1921, although he is known to have resented Husserl's attempt to claim him as one of his followers. Jaspers' phenomenology comes to the fore when he deals with the correlation of subject and object (for him, the fundamental phenomenon) and in his treatment of object-consciousness and ego-consciousness. In dealing with object-consciousness, for instance, he comes to recognise a 'phenomenological abyss' between the 'full-bodiedness' that characterises genuine hallucinations and the mere 'picture-likeness' that characterises illusory representations.

A contemporary of Jaspers and one very explicit in his embrace of phenomenology was the Swiss psychiatrist, Ludwig Binswanger. Binswanger was born into a family already distinguished for its service to medicine and psychiatry, his grandfather having established the Bellevue Sanatorium in Kreuzlingen. Binswanger became director of Bellevue after serving his internship in Zurich at the Burghölzli Mental Hospital, the foremost psychiatric clinic in Switzerland. Under Binswanger's director-ship, Bellevue became a meeting place for all kinds of scholars and artists. Among the philosophers who signed its guestbook were Max Scheler, Martin Heidegger and Martin Buber.

At the Burghölzli, Binswanger worked under Eugen Bleuler and Bleuler's then assistant, Carl Jung. In 1907 he accompanied Jung on a visit to Sigmund Freud in Vienna. This was for Binswanger the beginning of a firm friendship with Freud, contrasting with the turbulent relationship Freud had with Jung. Despite the friendship, Binswanger became ambivalent about Freudianism and felt a need for a philosophical anthropology that would keep the spotlight on human consciousness and biological processes together. From his original neo-Kantian philosophical background he moved through the life-philosophy of Dilthey and Bergson to a phenomenological stance based on Husserl, Scheler and Heidegger. For Binswanger, phenomenology offers access to the phenomena which his patients experience in their respective worlds. He comes to use Heidegger's concept of *Dasein* instead of Husserl's concept of con-sciousness and, in seeking an understanding of *Dasein*, he asserts that such knowledge must be grounded 'in the being together of me and you'. This leads Binswanger to a phenomenology of love. The love he focuses on is mutual love, especially romantic love, which issues in solidarity, a 'we-hood'. This is at variance with Heidegger's understanding of *Dasein* and Heidegger expressly rejected the use Binswanger made of his approach and terminology. In Heidegger's inquiry it is 'care' or 'concern' — an existential structure subsuming the many ways whereby the individual human being relates to entities in his or her world — that characterises existence most basically and most comprehensively. Binswanger sees things in another light. To him it is phenomenologically evident that love constitutes a basic structure of existence and that it is different from the 'care structure'. Love makes a difference to how people experience space and time and Binswanger proceeds to elucidate both aspects in his phenomenological inquiry.[27]

Binswanger led the way into phenomenology, and Heideggerian hermeneutics, for another Swiss psychiatrist, Medard Boss. Although he had been introduced to analysis by Sigmund Freud himself, had worked as Eugen Bleuler's assistant and studied with eminent practitioners such as Karen Horney, Wilhelm Reich and Carl Jung, Boss remained dissatisfied with the image of the human inherent in psychoanalysis.[28] Things changed for him when, inspired by Binswanger, Boss made contact with Heidegger and became his disciple and friend. Unlike Binswanger, Boss succeeded in winning Heidegger's approval for his approach and for many years Heidegger presented joint seminars with Boss in Switzerland.

Boss applies his phenomenological methods to such phenomena as sexual perversions, psychosomatic disturbances, and dreams. Where Freud takes for granted the structure of dreams as phenomena, Boss engages in a direct exploration of that structure. For him, the dream emerges as a way of 'being-there', *Dasein*, on a equal footing with wakefulness. His investigation of the dimensions of dreaming existence leads him to distinguish various kinds of dreams, to study the possibility of dreaming of dreaming, and even of analysing dreams while dreaming, and to draw out the structural differences between dream existence and wakeful existence. More recently Raymond McCall has attempted to find 'the best possible way to put the Boss-Heidegger position in American English' and to point up 'the possible impact of the Heidegger-Boss approach on the conceptual foundations of a contemporary psychology'.[29]

As Spiegelberg emphasises, many of the figures we have been considering here, and still others in the history of phenomenological psychology and psychiatry, have 'testified to the importance of phenomenological inspirations, confirmations, and corroborations in their research'.[30] They believe, undoubtedly, that their phenomenology has been fruitful.

Hopefully, this very selective account of their endeavours is able in some measure to convey the flavour of work done from this perspective. We have already had a taste of what is offered by the humanistic psychology which burgeoned in the United States in the early 1960s. The two are very different.

'Never the twain ...' ?

There are certainly affinities between the two psychologies and humanistic psychology as an organised movement has harboured, or at least claimed, a number of psychologists who espouse existential phenomenology. All the same, in a number of respects they make strange bed-fellows and in 1989 John Rowan publicly queried whether there are 'two humanistic psychologies or one'.[31]

By this time, as has been pointed out earlier, the textbooks were commonly singling out what they saw as the clear-cut distinguishing feature of humanistic psychology: the tenet that human beings are inherently growthful. According to this tenet, there is in all human beings a tendency to self-realisation — a notion deriving from Kurt Goldstein. For Goldstein, mentor to both Maslow and Rogers, existence is the condition in which individuals can actualize their essential capacities, or at least what they perceive to be their essential capacities. Maslow, Rogers and others made much of the notion of self-actualisation or self-realisation and it became emblematic for humanistic psychology. Rogers enunciates this notion in unmistakable terms:

Belief in the worth of the free person is not something that can be extinguished even by all the modern technological devices — bugging conversations, 'mental hospitals' to recondition behavior, electric tortures and all the rest. Nothing can extinguish the human organism's drive to be itself — to actualize itself in individual and creative ways.[32]

What Rowan had come to see was that this notion of an inherent tendency to self-actualisation is by no means common to all humanistic psychologists. There are psychologists, he wrote, who have to be seen as humanistic psychologists but whose thrust leads them, when considering issues of human fulfilment, to look to 'commitment', 'creativity', or 'personal action' rather than to some presumed innate drive towards positive growth. He is speaking of psychologists like Rollo May, Alvin Mahrer, and Ronald D Laing.

May admits that the human being is a bundle of potentialities. For him, however, these are 'the source of *both* our constructive and our destructive impulses'.[33] This was the very point that Martin Buber drove home to Carl Rogers in an historic colloquium at the University of Michigan in 1957. Using the example of a client, Rogers had stated that basic human nature 'is something that is really to be *trusted*' and that 'if we can release what is most basic in the individual, ... it will be constructive'. Buber's response was to point out that 'the good is always only a direction, not a substance'. What is called good and evil (Buber prefers 'yes and no', 'acceptance and refusal') are polarities. 'What you say may be trusted', he said to Rogers, 'stands in polar relation to what can be least trusted in this man.'[34]

These people whom Rowan singles out as departing from the textbook norm for the humanistic psychologist stand in the tradition of existential phenomenology. R D Laing, a British psychopathologist, was the co-founder of the Institute for Phenomenological Studies. The volume which May co-edited and contributed to in 1958, *Existence: A New Dimension in Psychiatry and Psychology*,[35] has been described by Spiegelberg as 'the most important event in the development of American phenomenological existentialism'.[36] Mahrer's excitingly different approach to therapy draws in part on the analysis of dreams effected by Medard Boss, whose phenomenological psychology has been referred to earlier in this chapter.

In some respects, Rowan suggests, psychologists such as Mahrer and May may be regarded as 'more narrowly and purely humanistic than Maslow and Rogers'. The irony of this is not lost on him, for he recognises that they are 'much less central' to the movement which Maslow and Rogers spearheaded. The point is that they are different and, if they are 'humanistic', theirs is a different brand of humanism. Mahrer has made this clear, setting out a 'case for fundamentally different existential-humanistic psychologies'.[37]

Spiegelberg too has highlighted the negligible part which those of a phenomenological bent have played in the context of the humanistic psychology movement in the United States. Maslow and Rogers have both been obviously sympathetic to phenomenology and both at times have used the term 'phenomenology' in relation to their own work. Nevertheless, neither can seriously be regarded as phenomenological in any true sense of the word. Referring to the masthead of the *Journal of Humanistic Psychology*, Spiegelberg states:

> 'Existential Psychology' and 'Phenomenological Psychology' are mentioned as congenial attempts to 'open up the vast and crucial inner life of man'. But as such they do not play a conspicuous part in the multifaceted activities of the 'Third Force'.[38]

In the United States, then, there have been few psychologists active within the humanistic psychology movement who attempt genuinely phenomenological inquiry. There are others who have worked outside its ambit and, throughout the 1960s, there was increasing interest in phenomenology within the American scene. Writing in 1972, Spiegelberg said of phenomenology in psychology:

> It will probably take much more time and effort before the new European ingredients have been critically absorbed and integrated into the mainstream of the American tradition.[39]

It is being suggested here that, instead of being absorbed and integrated, critically or otherwise, into the mainstream of the American tradition, the new European ingredients were assimilated to that tradition. This strange Continental mode of thought and inquiry was transposed into something more familiar, with humanistic psychology proving an effective instrument in this Americanising of phenomenology. Already part of the tradition referred to, humanistic psychology had succeeded in setting down deep roots and was not to be dislodged or even challenged.

Among the areas where humanistic psychology became so well established are the 'caring' or 'helping' professions such as nursing. Here it shows itself in an emphasis on a person-centred and holistic approach to health care. This can be found reflected in Munhall's table of 'expressions of contemporary nursing philosophy', which lists 'humanism', 'individualism', 'self-determinism', 'active organism', 'open system', 'holism', 'uniqueness', 'relativism', 'autonomy', 'advocacy' and 'organismic'.[40]

Yet, the rhetoric of phenomenology has also been appealing. Thus we find a marriage of phenomenological terminology with methods drawn from and based on the Maslow–Rogers form of humanistic psychology. This explains the anomaly often found in nursing literature and elsewhere where an unobjectionable exposition of phenomenology is coupled with a method that in no wise seeks to investigate phenomena but is content to deal with noetic aspects only in the style of humanistic psychology.

In all this, humanistic psychology has not stood alone. The interactionism of American social thought has had its impact too. And both have sprung from the matrix of a 'pragmatic-naturalist philosophy which focuses on the nature and genesis of a shared world, intersubjectivity, and communication'.[41] The kind of humanism found in humanistic psychology reflects the humanism of this heritage. It is a different humanism from that to be found in phenomenological psychology or, for that matter, phenomenological sociology and the other disciplinary areas where phenomenology has had impact.

Indeed, whether phenomenology as such can be regarded as humanistic is a moot point. Nursing phenomenologists have no qualms in labelling it so. Mason, one of those considered in Chapter 1, cites Bergum, another nurse researcher, in describing phenomenology as 'a humanistic science'.[42] Omery links the adoption of phenomenological methods in nursing to the intrinsic humanism of the profession and the discipline:

> The nursing profession is proud of its identification as a humanistic discipline. The profession's values and beliefs include a view that the human phenomenon is holistic and meaningful. The phenomenological methods share such values and beliefs.[43]

Thinkers who, like Heidegger, see phenomenology essentially as a method and philosophically without content would want to say that it cannot be described as humanistic. Pickles is following Heidegger when he claims that 'if it knows itself properly, phenomenology can never be a "humanism"'.[44]

Some would want to argue with this. As Thévenaz expresses it, 'what is originally conceived as a purely methodological innovation, without presuppositions, carries with it fundamental metaphysical options which sooner or later are bound to manifest themselves.'[45] In any case, even as methodology, it can be put to humanistic ends. That is precisely what Scheler is doing when he uses phenomenology to elaborate his philosophical anthropology. That is what the existential phenomenologists are doing when they wed phenomenological method to their various philosophies of existence.

As we have seen, Heidegger trenchantly dissociates himself from the humanism of Sartre's existentialism. However, just as he does not reject the tool of phenomenology which is in both Sartre's hands and his own, so too he does not reject humanism. It is just that his understanding of humanism differs radically from that embodied in Sartrean-style existentialism (and, as we have seen, from that espoused by nursing phenomenology). In fact, he will have no truck with any of the traditional forms of humanism because they 'all agree in this, that the *humanitas* of *homo humanus* is determined with regard to an already established interpretation of nature, history, world, and the ground of the world, that is, of beings as whole'. This, as Heidegger sees it, closes people off from the radical questioning of Being and the truth of Being. In that sense, humanism in its traditional forms emerges as anti-humanism. It not only fails to ask the question about the relation of Being to human being, but 'even impedes the question by neither recognizing nor understanding it'.[46] Heidegger rejects any humanism that would make the human person 'the Lord of beings' instead of 'the shepherd of Being'. Rather than lordship of beings, there is nearness to Being. Each of us, says Heidegger, is 'the neighbour of Being'.

> Is this not 'humanism' in the extreme sense? Certainly. It is humanism that thinks the humanity of man from nearness to Being. But at the same time it is a humanism in which not man but man's historical essence is at stake in its provenance from the truth of Being.[47]

Levin sums up Heidegger's position:

> For Heidegger, we must break away from the self-centredness of our tradition, a humanism which, since the beginning of modernity, has conceived the 'Self' of this centredness in terms of egoity; and we must begin to question ourselves in terms of a 'Self' centred, instead, by its (decentring) openness to Being.[48]

For all his strictures against Sartre, Heidegger's view of human beings as beings-in-the-world is one that he shares with the whole tradition of existential phenomenology. The humanism of the existential phenomenologists has not been guilty of conceiving the self 'in terms of egoity', as Levin puts it. It has refused to dichotomise subject and object but instead has pointed to an indissoluble union between people and their worlds. Even Husserl, for all his idealism, addresses not an isolated self but life-experiencing-the-world. It is hard to level an accusation of self-centredness against a humanism of this kind.

The same cannot be said of the humanism of humanistic psychology. The accusation of excessive self-centredness and subjectivism has been made many times over. As early as 1973, Misiak and Sexton were reporting the concern of various members of the humanistic movement about 'the "increasing slippage" between the idealism of humanistic psychology and reality'. They also reported this comment of Heinz Ansbacher about humanistic psychology:

> By its emphasis on the self and absence of the concept of social usefulness, it has recently tended to attract self-seeking groups to the dismay of its responsible leaders. By adopting the concept of social interest the movement would have a tool to remedy the situation and to find a clearer definition of its purpose and direction.[49]

While Ansbacher uses the term 'self-seeking', this is not to be read in the pejorative sense it tends to conjure up. The groups to which he refers are not being accused of egoism or selfishness or self-indulgence. They are groups, rather, whose members are in search of their own selves. A laudable aim, and one that can be linked to the age-old Socratic injunction, 'Know thyself!'. But, if not egoistic, these groups can be seen as egocentric. They are focused on the growth and development of the self conceived in a highly individualistic fashion. Interpersonal relations may be highlighted, it is true, but these tend to be seen as serving an instrumental function, i.e. they are important for the actualisation of the self. This is the basic orientation of the human potential movement which burgeoned in the United States in the 1960s, starting from California. Almost from the start it seized upon humanistic psychology and developed alongside it. Writing of 'the birth of the Esalen Institute in the 1960s and the legacy it has left to the new age movement', Ted Peters points to the role of leading humanistic psychologists:

> In the summer of 1962 connection was made with Abraham Maslow. Maslow, along with Carl Rogers, was the intellectual architect of the human potential movement. Rogers had given us the term *self-realization*, and Maslow *self-actualization*.[50]

Peters goes on to highlight the contribution of Fritz Perls, Will Schutz and psychosynthesist Robert Assagioli. Assagioli took the search for self to another level, offering a method of getting in touch with the 'higher self'. In this way, Peters points out, the human potential movement moved 'beyond personal and interpersonal relations into transpersonal or metaphysical psychology'. So too did some sections of the humanistic psychology movement, as later contents of the *Journal of Humanistic Psychology* attest.

The 'dismay' which Ansbacher speaks of is still experienced in some quarters. Writing in the *Journal of Humanistic Psychology*, Associate Editor Maureen O'Hara[51] points to 'epistemological confusion' within the humanistic psychologies and to their 'overemphasis on the individual self'. She considers the 'view of the person as an autonomous center of consciousness as proposed by humanistic psychologists' to be an illusion, reminding us that 'our autonomous sense of a private, unique self *is given to us by our culture*', i.e. it 'comes to us from outside'. This, she asserts, is not acknowledged by humanistic psychology. We need to acknowledge it, for 'we pay a high price for our illusion of autonomy'.

> It is an illusion that abstracts us from the intersubjective reality of our relationships to culture, traditions, history, institutions, families and communities, and especially to each other. It sets an idealized 'unencumbered self' *against* the world that gives it life, breath and, especially, meaning.[52]

The 'reality' of these relationships is the insight we have seen Benner expressing when she describes our freedom as 'situated'. Unfortunately, she proceeds in large measure to distance herself from the implications of this 'situated freedom' as entailing a hermeneutics of suspicion. It is a crucial insight, nonetheless, and should be accorded the emphasis it deserves. To the extent that a genuinely phenomenological perspective sets the person *in* the world and not against the world, it may be seen as offering a welcome counterbalance to the kind of subjectivism for which humanistic psychology is criticised. In Chapter 3 above, we noted the warning of Merleau-Ponty not to seek truth within us as if it inhabited some inner self. There is, he states baldly, *no* inner self. Instead, we are in the world and it is only in the world that we know ourselves. Each of us, he reminds us, is 'a subject destined to be in the world'.[53] If philosophy, as the search for truth, can be said at all to bring us back to an 'interior', the interior it brings us to is 'not a "private life" but an intersubjectivity that gradually connects us ever closer to the whole of history'.[54]

In short, nurse researchers need not fear that the outcomes of research would be less humanistic if they were to move from an approach informed by the humanism of humanistic psychology to one grounded in authentic phenomenology. In any case, it is not being suggested that they make that move in some sort of definitive and exclusive fashion. It is not a question of either-or. Phenomenology seeks an intentional analysis that embraces *both* object and subject, the noematic and the noetic. The noematic elements — the phenomena — may be primary, but they are discovered within the field of human consciousness and experience. The study of the objects of experience and the study of the experiencing subject proceed hand in hand. What an investigation in the spirit of existential phen-omenology would ensure is that experiencing subjects are not divorced from their worlds. It would keep the spotlight on their intrinsic relatedness, i.e. on their being-in-the-world and their being-with-others.

This brings to the fore the sociality that lies at the core of our being. We are, says Merleau-Ponty, 'through and through compounded of relationships with the world.'[55]

> As long as I cling to the ideal of an absolute spectator, of knowledge with no point of view, I can see my situation as nothing but a source of error. But if I have once recognized that through it I am grafted onto every action and all knowledge which can have a meaning for me, and that step by step it contains everything that can *exist* for me, then my contact with the social in the finitude of my situation is revealed to me as the point of origin of all truth, including scientific truth.[56]

My contact with the social as the point of origin of all truth. It is time to consider the contribution of phenomenological sociology.

NOTES

1 'For Scheler, phenomenology was an "attitude" based in a "psychic technique of non resistance", a special act of spirit that blocks the normal flow of life to reveal its growing, striving becoming tendencies, on the one side, and the givenness of the world as resistance, on the other ...'
'To begin with, phenomenology for Scheler was not a method, as it was for Husserl, but an "attitude of spiritual seeing", because "A method is a goal-directed procedure of *thinking about* facts, for example, induction or deduction. In phenomenology, however, it is a matter first, of new facts themselves, before they have been fixed by logic, and second, of a procedure of *seeing*".' (Stikkers 1985, pp. 129–130)
2 See Scheler (1974ff).
3 Cited in Emad (1972), p. 361.
4 *Ibid.*, p. 369.
5 *Ibid.*, p. 370.
6 Moore (1965), p. 95.
7 See Heron (1970).
8 Buber (1958), p. 97.
9 Heron (1970), p. 264.
10 Rogers (1961), p. 53.
11 *Ibid.*, p. 61.
12 *Ibid.*, p. 18.
13 *Ibid.*, p. 34.
14 Dobbie (1991), p. 826.
15 See Rogers (1969).
16 See Arnett and Nakagawa (1983).
17 This unquestioning acceptance of what others say of themselves is not reflected in mainstream phenomenology. 'I must not succumb to the naive position (as Bittner hints as being the source of the problem of an abortive phenomenology) of accepting the statements respondents make as the literal and sufficient explanations of their conduct, beliefs, values and knowledge.' (Psathas 1973, pp. 15–16)
18 Benner and Wrubel (1989), p. 57.
19 Rose (1990), p. 60.
20 Dobbie (1991), p. 826. The reference is to Massarik (1981), p. 203.
21 Rose (1990), p. 60.
22 Wood (1991), p. 196.
23 See Maslow (1957).
24 Cited in Misiak and Sexton (1973), p. 116.
25 See Spiegelberg (1972), pp. 42–52.
26 *Ibid.*, p. 191.
27 For examples of Binswanger's phenomenology, see Binswanger (1963). Also see May, Angel and Ellenberger (1958), pp. 191–364.
28 See McCall (1983), Introduction.
29 *Ibid.*, pp. 4, 96.
30 Spiegelberg (1972), pp. 361–362.
31 See Rowan (1989).
32 Rogers (1978), p. 261.
33 May (1982), p. 11.
34 See Buber (1966), pp. 179–181.
35 See May, Angel and Ellenberger (1958).

36 Spiegelberg (1972), p. 163.
37 See Mahrer (1989).
38 Spiegelberg (1972), p. 167.
39 *Ibid*, p. 168.
40 Munhall (1982), p. 177. The table referred to is reprinted in Munhall and Oiler (1986), p. 21.
41 Rogers (1981), p. 140.
42 Mason (1992), p. 556.
43 Omery (1983), p. 62.
44 Pickles (1985), p. 50.
45 Thévenaz (1962), p. 38.
46 Heidegger (1977b), p. 202.
47 *Ibid*., pp. 221–222.
48 Levin (1989), p. 64.
49 Misiak and Sexton (1973), p. 127.
50 Peters (1991), p. 12.
51 See O'Hara (1989).
52 *Ibid*., p. 270.
53 Merleau-Ponty (1962), p. xi.
54 Merleau-Ponty (1964b), p. 112.
55 Merleau-Ponty (1962), p. xiii.
56 Merleau-Ponty (1964b), p. 109.

6

Phenomenology and the social world

Nursing research rarely attempts to draw on phenomenological sociology. None of the thirty pieces of research considered in Chapter 1 can be said to do so to any real extent. In nursing research there is the odd reference to Alfred Schutz, from time to time an invoking of ethnomethodology, and some talk of 'shared meanings and common practices'. However, most nurse researchers seeking to follow a phenomenological path tend to remain psychological in their orientation.

Phenomenological sociology is by no means easy to grapple with. Even in its origins phenomenological sociology is complex and obscure. Those origins are commonly seen to lie within the work of Alfred Schutz,[1] whose views bring together a number of traditions. These include Husserlian phenomenology but also Weberianism and American interactionism (not to speak of a Kantian element here and there).

Nurse researchers would not be greatly helped in this respect by the available sociology textbooks. Most of these texts ignore phenomenology as such. A few give some consideration to ethnomethodology. Anthony Giddens' *Sociology* published in 1989 is a case in point. The word 'phenomenology' is not to be found in either its 'Glossary of basic concepts' or its 'Glossary of important terms', nor does the word seem to occur in the text. Ethnomethodology is given a definition (a somewhat dubious one at that) in the second of the glossaries referred to and has some four pages of text devoted to it. John J Macionis's *Sociology* is another example: it too ignores phenomenology while offering a definition and a less-than-one-page explanation of ethnomethodology.

Misreading of phenomenology

Those texts that do talk of phenomenology commonly confuse it with interpretative sociology in general[2] or identify it with social constructionism, positing as its main interest something like Macionis' (misleading) definition of ethnomethodology: 'the study of the everyday, commonsense understandings that people have of the world around them'.[3] It is a commonplace to see phenomenology in sociology described as an approach which emphasises the social construction of reality and is concerned with exploring people's shared perceptions and meanings. In this vein, as we have seen in an earlier chapter, Patricia Benner's 'Heideggerian phenomenology' looks to 'a shared background of common meanings'.[4] Benner's approach is endorsed by Diekelmann, one of the authors analysed at the start of this book:

> Heideggerian hermeneutics, first introduced to nursing by Benner, seeks to reveal the frequently taken for granted shared practices and common meanings embedded in our day-to-day lived experiences ... [5]

As has been contended throughout this study, this is not phenomenology. It is a form of social inquiry that is in continuity with the American intellectual tradition but owes nothing to the phenomenological movement. It relates to the symbolic interactionism emanating from the thought of George Herbert Mead rather than to phenomenology, whether transcendental or existentialist. J Clyde Mitchell writes of this kind of sociological exploration:

> Some interpretive sociologists — those identified as 'symbolic interactionists' for example — are content to operate with a relatively naïve set of assumptions about how we come to know about social phenomena. They are prepared to accept the meanings that the actors attribute to social phenomena at face value, and proceed to erect their systematic interpretations on these foundations. This implies that the sociological observer must exercise sufficient discipline on himself to ensure that it is indeed the *actors*' meanings that are recorded in his notebook and not merely his own.[6]

This seeking of 'the meanings that the actors attribute to social phenomena at face value', all the while striving to ensure that they are the actors' meanings and not meanings imposed on the data by the investigator, is precisely the process put forward as phenomenology by the new phenomenologists. Yet Mitchell, quite rightly, attributes such a process not to phenomenology but to forms of interpretative sociology such as symbolic interactionism.

We find Denzin[7] similarly pointing out that the social construction of reality is one of the 'primitive assumptions' of symbolic interactionism.

'Reality', he writes of this point of view, 'as it is sensed, known and understood is a social production.' Hence the need to see things as the social actors themselves see it. 'Methodologically, symbolic interactionism directs the investigator to take, to the best of his ability, the standpoint of those studied.'

Psathas too attributes this approach not to phenomenology but to symbolic interactionism.

> Methodologically, the implication of the symbolic interactionist perspective is that the actor's view of actions, objects, and society has to be studied seriously. The situation must be seen as the actor sees it, the meanings of objects and acts must be determined in terms of the actor's meanings, and the organization of a course of action must be understood as the actor organizes it. The role of the actor in the situation would have to be taken by the observer in order to see the social world from his perspective.[8]

If we return to Mitchell, we read that, while 'it is important to understand "how the world looks" to those who live in it' there are sociologists who believe that 'this does not go far enough'.[9] These 'critics', as he calls them, are not content to explore the understandings which members of society have of their world but want to examine *how* they come to have such understandings.

Phenomenologists are among these critics. As it happens, the example Mitchell gives of their work is a study of juvenile delinquency by Cicourel,[10] who, significantly, is closely identified with phenomenology and a particular form of ethnomethodology. Phenomenologists are in the vanguard of those who insist that it is not enough to explore the sense that people make of their world, but require that we look to how that understanding of the world comes into being for them.

Nevertheless, a concern with the genesis of social meanings is still not enough in itself to put the stamp of phenomenology on social investigation. A piece of social inquiry may explore how understandings of the world have been constructed but what determines whether or not it is phenomenological inquiry is the manner in which the investigation is conducted and not merely the fact that it takes place. Phenomenologists carry out such inquiry by looking to the original encounter of subject with object, seeking, as it were, to re-experience that encounter so that its possibilities for meaning may emerge afresh. To do that requires a bracketing of the everyday assumptions of the natural attitude. 'Bracketing', says Psathas, 'changes my attitude towards the world, allowing me to see with clearer vision.' More than that, when the researcher sets aside preconceptions and presuppositions and examines the world anew precisely 'as it is experienced', a whole range of experiences become objects of attention and study that would ordinarily have been passed over. In a phenomenological approach to the social world, Psathas is thus able to claim, the inquirer is in a position both 'to discover it with clarity of vision' and 'to expand his view'.[11]

So phenomenology requires a bracketing of prevailing and inherited understandings rather than an exploration of these understandings and their social generation. Instead of seeing shared meanings as a straightforward path to insight about social reality, phenomenologists suspect that they also serve as a blindfold. In this vein, Kurt Wolff writes of Schutz's 'world of paramount reality' — the *Lebenswelt* — and offers a salutary warning:

> If we, sociologists or not, but we sociologists too, trust our senses, rather than the received notions that blind them, and thus us, to reality, the only way we can begin coming to terms with our 'paramount reality' is to say No to it, for, as Herbert Marcuse put it, '"The whole is the truth" and the whole is false'.[12]

This, Wolff goes on to say, is to advocate 'suspending (not rejecting nor affirming) one's traditions as best one can'. Here we have the phenomenological endeavour to get behind 'received notions' and 'shared meanings' so as to address the phenomena that underlie them. 'Back to the things themselves!'

The overlooking of this essential dimension of phenomenological inquiry constitutes, it may be suggested, a 'hijacking' of phenomenological discourse by more traditionally American lines of thought. Here phenomenology comes to be identified with symbolic interactionism and the social constructionism inherent in both. Jack D Douglas writes explicitly in this vein:

> Because of its rejection of an absolutist view of social problems, the interactionist theory is the first example of what we can call a *phenomenological theory of social problems*. All phenomenological theories share four basic ideas about social problems: (1) *the sociologist must first study social problems and their solutions from the standpoints of the members of society*; (2) when the sociologist does study social problems in this way he finds that *the meanings of social problems to the members of our society are highly problematic*; (3) the problematic nature of social problems means that *there will be basic conflicts among the members of society in defining social problems*; and (4) these conflicts mean that *the sociologist who is committed to providing objective and practically useful information and explanations of those social problems must analyze the ways in which conflicting groups construct the meanings of social problems and solutions to those problems*.[13]

Douglas believes that this discovery of 'problems' within the meanings adhered to by members of society, leading to an exploration of how the members construct their 'meanings and paths of action', is what characterises phenomenological sociology.

> The phenomenological analyses of social meanings and actions in general have revealed that these problems of meaning make it necessary for the members of society to *construct specific, concrete meanings and paths of actions for each concrete situation they face in everyday life*. That is, the members must put together specific interpretations of their shared meanings (values, beliefs, ideas, feelings) that seem to them to be relevant and plausible for the situations at hand. Also, as one would expect, the more problematic the meanings applied to any concrete situation are, the more *constructive or interpretive work* the members must do to construct plausible, acceptable meanings to deal with that situation. Much of phenomenological sociology has been concerned with showing how they go about doing this, especially with showing what leads to one construction of meaning and action rather than to others.[14]

While phenomenologists would have no great problem with any of Douglas' four tenets, none of them is the hallmark of phenomenology. A number of clearly non-phenomenological approaches embrace these same principles. Moreover, phenomenology does not find its primary focus in the contradictions and conflict discernible in people's interpretation of their everyday world. To the contrary, its focus is precisely those aspects of social understanding that appear uncontrovertible — the taken-for-granted features. Far from seizing upon that which is problematic, phenomenology takes what is unproblematic and problematises it. It involves, Natanson tells us, a 'transformation of familiarity into strangeness'.[15] Such transformation is brought about by holding our taken-for-granted understandings in abeyance and taking a fresh look at the phenomena to which they attach.

Alfred Schutz did precisely that with what he liked to term the 'commonsense world'. He engaged in a phenomenology of the everyday world which we all experience and which is for us, he said, our 'paramount reality'.

The work of Alfred Schutz

Schutz (1899–1959) was born in Vienna. After military service during World War I, he studied law and economics at the University of Vienna. However, he was not to be a typical academic and that was made clear very early. Even before gaining his doctorate, he had taken up an advisory position with a consortium of Viennese banks. This was the kind of employment that would provide him with a livelihood in the United States also, when he went there in 1939. Of Jewish descent, Schutz left Austria as a refugee when the Nazi powers occupied the country. In New York, he joined the New School of Social Research but his academic work was done outside of normal working hours. By day during the week he was a banking consultant. He became a full-time academic for the first time just two and a half years before his death in 1959.

Some seven years before leaving Europe to settle in America, Schutz had published *Der sinnhafte Aufbau der sozialen Welt*, which appeared in English in 1967 as *The Phenomenology of the Social World*. In a lifetime of writing, this was the one and only full-length book he published. Many of his writings were published posthumously in *Collected Papers I-III* (1962–1966) and in 1973 *The Structure of the Life-World* appeared with Thomas Luckmann as co-author.

The Phenomenology of the Social World reflects a twofold influence on Schutz during his time at the University of Vienna. There he had come into contact with the sociology of Weber, who had lectured at that university in 1918, and the philosophy of Husserl, with whom he was to have an enduring personal friendship. Schutz's commitment to phenomenology, which emerged from this involvement with Husserl and Husserlian thought, was strengthened by meetings with Maurice Merleau-Ponty and Raymond Aron during a year he spent as a refugee in France before moving to the United States.

For all that, it was Weber who remained central to Schutz's emerging methodology. Schutz had the utmost respect for Weber's work, especially his goal of value-neutrality, his concept of '*verstehen* sociology' (a sociology of action and understanding, with emphasis on social actors' motivations and meanings) and his use of 'ideal types'. The task Schutz set himself was to provide a philosophical grounding for Weber's approach to social inquiry, which was something Weber himself had failed to do. After looking in vain to Bergson's philosophy for such a foundation, Schutz turned to Husserl.

Max Weber introduces his 'ideal type' as a conceptual tool for social analysis. The problem Weber is addressing is one that had loomed large in German social thought for some time, being a preoccupation with thinkers such as Dilthey, Windelband and Rickert. The basic issue is how the social interaction of free, self-conscious actors can be examined scientifically. Their individual actions, the very stuff of human history, make up the subject matter of any study of society. How applicable to this kind of subject matter are the methods of natural science? Hence the dilemma that all social scientists are seen to be facing — of the general *versus* the particular, the nomothetic over against the idiographic. If social scientists are content with general concepts in explaining social situations, they are likely to overlook features that are most distinctive of those situations. If their account of social phenomena is totally particularised, it becomes impossible to compare these with other, even similar, phenomena. The ideal type is introduced by Weber as a way out of this impasse.

Weber's *verstehen* ('understanding') sociology locates the study of society in the context of human beings acting and interacting.

> Interpretative sociology considers the individual and his action as the basic unit, as its 'atom' ... The individual is ... the upper limit and the sole carrier of meaningful conduct ... Such concepts as 'state', 'association', 'feudalism', and the like, designate certain categories of human interaction. Hence it is the task of sociology to reduce these concepts to 'understandable' action, that is without exception, to the actions of participating men.[16]

Weber feels the need to focus social inquiry on the meanings and values of individual acting persons and therefore on their subjective 'meaning-complex of action'. He defines sociology as a science which attempts to understand social action interpretatively so as to arrive at a causal explanation of its course and its effects.[17] For him, as far as human affairs are concerned, any understanding of causation comes through an interpretative understanding of social action involving an explanation of relevant antecedent phenomena as meaning-complexes. Here the outcomes are different from those pursued in the natural sciences. The causation that the social scientist seeks to clarify is at best 'adequate' rather than 'necessary'.

At the same time, it is Weber's contention that, in any scientific study of society, *verstehen* has to be substantiated by empirical evidence. He has a passion for empirical knowledge and stresses the need for scientifically valid historical and social data. Weber's philosophy, Lewis assures us, is 'an empiricist venture'.

> It was as strictly an empirical sociology as academic philosophy was speculative. For it attempted to establish a science of social fact, and to use an appropriate methodology devised for historico-political material rather than for the natural sciences, a methodology which would describe and classify historical and social facts schematically and deduce experimentally the laws-system of society.[18]

Weber finds the centrepiece of this 'appropriate methodology' in what he calls the ideal type. This is his principal diagnostic tool, a heuristic device for the precise purpose of amassing empirical data. It seeks to subject social behaviour, essentially subjective as it is, to the scientific need for the empirical verification of all knowledge.

Using the word 'tool' to describe Weber's ideal type points up the important fact that it is a human construct. It is something the social scientist makes up and not something found through an analysis of what is real. What it embodies is the 'pure case', with no admixture of

135

adventitious and confusing features. As such, it never exists in reality, but can serve as a useful model which guides the social inquirer in addressing the real-life case and discerning where and to what extent the real deviates from the ideal.

Weber sets strict limits to the use of his ideal types. He believes that ideal-type methodology is applicable only to social behaviour that can be described as 'rational goal-oriented conduct' and not to 'rational value-oriented conduct', 'affectual conduct', or 'traditionalist conduct'. What is being studied by way of the ideal type is seen to be the outcome of persons acting under a common motivation and choosing suitable means to the ends they have in view. It is only in regard to such rational goal-oriented conduct that we can take stock of empirical data according to preconceived rational criteria implicitly accepted by both actor and observer.

Alfred Schutz was very taken with Weber's ideal-type methodology. However, more of a philosopher than Weber, he recognised that Weber uses terms like 'understanding' and 'meaning', and indeed makes them the linchpin of his approach to social science, without ever establishing or elucidating them as concepts. He does not found 'a meaning for meaning' and has no theory of subjectivity to offer. For this reason, as Schutz sees it, Weber's talk of value-relevance, *verstehen* and even ideal typification becomes unclear and unscientific. Without such grounding, how can anyone create ideal types that genuinely reflect the meanings of typical actors in typical circumstances? Without such grounding, it surely becomes just a matter of guesswork.

Schutz's goal, therefore, is to 'give to interpretive sociology the philosophical basis it has hitherto lacked'.[19] He intends to provide a valid philosophical grounding for Weber's 'subjectivity' and the associated terms he uses such as 'meaning', 'understanding', 'motivation' and 'action'. To do this, he draws upon Husserl and phenomenology and engages in a phenomenological description of the lifeworld. At the time of writing *The Phenomenology of the Social World*, he accepted in principle the notion of Husserl's transcendental reduction, although over the years he came to regard it as unnecessary for the philosophical grounding of intersubjectivity.

> ... intersubjectivity is not a problem of constitution which can be solved within the transcendental sphere, but is rather a datum ... of the life-world. It is the fundamental ontological category of human existence in the world and therefore of all philosophical anthropology.[20]

Even in *The Phenomenology of the Social World* Schutz moves at once from the transcendental realm attained by the phenomenological reduction back to the commonsense world of everyday life.

> ... our analysis will be carried out within the phenomenological reduction only so far as this is necessary for acquiring a clear understanding of the internal time-consciousness.

The purpose of this work, which is to analyze the phenomenon of meaning in ordinary (*mundanen*) social life, does not require the achievement of a transcendental knowledge that goes beyond that sphere or a further sojourn within the area of the transcendental-phenomenological reduction. In ordinary social life we are no longer concerned with the constituting phenomena as these are studied within the sphere of the phenomenological reduction. We are concerned only with the phenomena corresponding to them within the natural attitude.[21]

Schutz, then, addresses the life-world in phenomenological fashion, trying to get behind the taken-for-granted world of everyday life. Beneath the meanings attaching to this world he seeks the way in which meaning is constituted through what he calls the 'operating intentionality of an Ego-consciousness'.[22] He is led to a description of this Ego-consciousness and its inner time. He finds himself led along 'with others' and therefore led to intersubjectivity. He is concerned with meaning and is therefore led to relevances.

In and out of all of this there emerges for him the insight that in the commonsense world actors behave on the basis of typifications. It is true that we are all unique persons, each coming from a different 'biographical situation'. It is also true that we perceive the world and make it our own within this biographical situation. As we do so, however, we bring to bear a 'stock of knowledge at hand', which consists of a set of socially derived and socially approved typifications. These serve as 'social recipes' which enable us to act in typical ways in given circumstances and to expect typical outcomes.

For Schutz, typifications used in the social sciences derive from these typifications of daily life and are patterned upon them. This leads him to the notion of second-order ideal-type constructs mirroring the real-life typifications which actually influence social actors and explain typical social interaction. These second-order types Schutz refers to as *homunculi* or 'puppets'. The *homunculi* can serve as instruments for an inductive derivation of empirical facts. In other words, we can check them against empirical reality and verify them or amend them.

True enough, these ideal-type models — the 'puppets' — are constructs of the social scientist. According to Schutz, the *homunculus*

> ... does not assume a role other than that attributed to him by the director of the puppet show ... It is he, the social scientist, who sets the stage, who distributes the role, who gives the cues, who defines when an 'action' starts and when it ends and who determines, thus, the 'span of projects' involved. All standards and institutions governing the behavioral pattern of the model are supplied from the outset by the constructs of the scientific observer.[23]

The social scientist, nonetheless, cannot set the stage and distribute roles arbitrarily. The *homunculi* need to meet certain criteria:

* *the postulate of logical consistency*
  The model must be clear and compatible with logical principles so as to make sense to the social scientists using it.
* *the postulate of subjective interpretation*
  The model must refer human action and its outcomes to the subjective meanings they hold for the social actors.
* *the postulate of adequacy*
  There needs to be consistency between the scientist's constructs and the typifications to be found in commonsense experience of social reality. The model must be able to explain how the act to which it refers would be understood by the actor and those with whom the actor interacts if it took place in real life.

If they conform to such principles, despite their 'artificial' character, *homunculi* can serve effectively in their intended role.

All this is Weberianism revisited, but Schutz believes that, through his use of phenomenological inquiry, he has done what Weber failed to do and has grounded his system epistemologically.

Phenomenology and sociology

Whether Schutz does provide a valid grounding for his methodology is much debated. Questions are also raised about the kind of freedom Schutz's methodology allows for. His grounding of subjectivity and intersubjectivity, it is asserted, only succeeds, if it succeeds in anything, in reducing human freedom to the ability to behave 'freely' in typical, socially prescribed ways. 'What kind of freedom is that?', the critics ask. Few of them find their misgivings allayed by Schutz's distinction between 'because-motives' and 'in-order-to-motives' or his description of how these are supposed to interlock in the course of social interaction.

Such criticism apart, Schutz is clearly not offering a phenomenological sociology in any substantive sense.

Schutz certainly uses phenomenology to establish his method. He invokes a phenomenological reduction to do so. An interesting version of it, as it happens, for, where Husserl talks of suspending belief, Schutz talks of suspending doubt. It is his view that in the natural attitude people already engage in an *epoché*: they put in brackets any doubt that the world may not be as it appears to be.

> Phenomenology has taught us the concept of phenomenological *epoché*, the suspension of our belief in the reality of the world as a device to overcome the natural attitude by radicalizing the Cartesian method of

philosophical doubt. The suggestion may be ventured that man within the natural attitude also uses a specific *epoché*, of course quite another one than the phenomenologist. He does not suspend belief in the outer world and its objects, but on the contrary, he suspends doubt in its existence. What he puts in brackets is the doubt that the world and its objects might be otherwise than it appears to him. We propose to call this *epoché* the *epoché of the natural attitude*.[24]

What Schutz proposes is an *epoché* of this *epoché* already carried out in the natural attitude. He suggests that this habitual suspension of doubt about the reality of our world be brought to an end. The commonsense world may constitute our 'paramount reality' but, to proceed phenomenologically, we need to lay aside the understandings we have of it. We must doubt systematically all that this commonsense world takes for granted. That is what Schutz attempts to do.

His phenomenological inquiry leads him to analyses of typifications and social recipes, as we have seen. It leads him also to insights into 'projects of action', a categorisation of our fellow humans ('predecessors', 'contemporaries', 'consociates', 'successors'), and the notion of 'multiple realities' that exist for them and for us. This exposition has been described by Natanson[25] as 'an anatomy of typifications of social reality' and 'an inventory of phenomenological machinery'.

What if one wants more? Natanson deals with that question. What if one 'wants to know something of the nature of "directly experienced social reality"? What if one wants 'an elucidation of the originary situation'? Natanson believes that, in terms of social reality, 'the "directly experienced" yields to phenomenological description' and that Schutz's analysis has something to offer in this respect. We are able to inquire phenomenologically into the 'givenness of sociality' and Schutz can assist us in the task.

While Schutz uses phenomenology to establish the tool he sees as necessary for social inquiry and while Schutzian phenomenology may elucidate the meaning of sociality itself, social inquiry carried out through use of the tool and in terms of that elucidation is not in itself phenomenological. We are still far from a phenomenological sociology whose substance derives from phenomenological inquiry. It is very doubtful whether Schutz believes such a sociology is possible.

If a substantive phenomenological sociology is possible, phenomenology emerges as a rival to other forms of sociology. It can be seen, in Grossberg's terms,[26] as a challenge *for* sociology, which has to accommodate it. In a sense, Schutz's project is an even greater challenge, for it arrogates to phenomenology the task of developing sociology's very tools. As Grossberg says of another attempt to 'derive or explicate ... sociological methods from the phenomenological method',[27] this can be seen as an attempt by phenomenology to dominate sociology and therefore as a challenge *to* sociology.

There are other ways in which phenomenology can be a challenge to sociology. Grossberg talks of attempts to find in phenomenology — and specifically in existential-ontological phenomenology — a framework which would enable scientific sociological findings to be related to the general structures of human existence. Phenomenology can be seen, in fact, to have a genuinely critical role *vis-à-vis* the achievements of science: 'to challenge the pretensions of science, to debunk the latter's claim to provide a full or even an adequate understanding of human life'.[28]

Yet another challenge to sociology pointed up by Grossberg is that of ethnomethodology. Its acknowledged founder is Harold Garfinkel, although over the years ethnomethodology has assumed several forms, some of which are in marked contrast to Garfinkel's version of it. For Garfinkel, for instance, there is 'nothing of interest under the skull' whereas, in Aaron Cicourel's ethnomethodology, 'it is in understanding the minds of persons that one finds the keystone of how social behavior unfolds'.[29]

Garfinkel was led by his interest in Schutz and other phenomenologists to an analysis of the structure of the everyday world. A group of colleagues and students formed around him and in 1967 he published *Studies in Ethnomethodology*. The everyday world on which Garfinkel focuses is characterised by consistency, coherence, planfulness, method and reproducibility. Such characteristics are what Garfinkel calls the 'rational properties' of social acts and social occasions. They are not, however, to be seen as intrinsic properties. Rather, such features stem from ongoing effort on the part of members of society. The members (a term that ethnomethodologists like to use) work hard to make their world appear organised and accountable. They have their own ways of deciding such properties, recognising them, and making them accountable to themselves. Accounts of such 'methods', revealed in members' behaviour (*ethno*-methods, therefore, since they belong to the 'people' or the 'folk'), form the focal point of ethnomethodological investigation. Ethnomethodology seeks to identify the processes whereby members, in any given social setting, make such features as consistency and orderliness visible, demonstrable and accountable. In doing so, it seeks to identify the basic properties of these processes.

Coherence, consistency and order are taken for granted in everyday life, but ethnomethodology does not take them for granted. It calls them into question. Here ethnomethodologists have their own form of the phenomenological reduction. They put in brackets all beliefs and understandings about the everyday world except the practices which members use to produce and maintain the setting as something undestandable, consistent and accountable. These practices are the phenomena that ethnomethodology explores and wants to explain.

Ethnomethodology has been a sign of contradiction since its emergence in the 1960s. There are those who want to say that it is not phenomenology. Indeed, there are those who want to say that it is not even sociology.[30]

Some want to extend the same sort of criticism to the work of Alfred Schutz from which ethnomethodology draws its inspiration.

That assessment of the Schutzian project and of ethnomethodology is not endorsed here. It is true that neither Schutz's work nor ethnomethodology represents Husserlian phenomenology, but neither claims to be doing that. Zygmunt Bauman is therefore overstating his case and overlooking the astonishing diversity of the phenomenological movement when he writes:

> It took guile, utterly illegitimate from the Husserlian perspective, to devise a social science which could claim to be the brainchild, or logical consequence of the phenomenological project.[31]

It is also true that the prevailing currents of American thought had their impact on Schutz, Garfinkel and their followers. Jonathan Turner writes of 'the phenomenological-interactionism of Alfred Schutz' and considers that Schutz's contribution 'resides in his ability to blend Husserl's radical phenomenology with Max Weber's action theory and American interactionism'.[32] Ethnomethodology, Turner also claims, 'borrows and extends ideas from phenomenology and, despite disclaimers to the contrary, from Meadian-inspired symbolic interactionism'.[33]

Nevertheless, it must be said that both Schutz and the ethnomethodologists follow the phenomenological path. As has been pointed out, Schutz does so, not to found a phenomenological sociology in the true sense of the term, but to ground his methodology for what remains essentially a Weberian project. In doing so, he uses a phenomenological reduction. While this may not be the transcendental reduction of Edmund Husserl, it represents, nonetheless, a genuine attempt to get behind the everyday, taken-for-granted meanings of the commonsense world.

The same is true of ethnomethodology. It seeks to get behind our everyday acceptance of social order and consistency so as to bring into focus the methods members of society use to create the *sense* that there is coherence, planfulness, orderliness and reproducibility in the world they experience.

It is in this way that Schutzian and ethnomethodological approaches to social reality differ from, say, symbolic interactionism or ethnographic methods. For these latter, everyday accounts are a resource. For phenomenology, however, to use the terminology employed by Zimmerman and Pollner in expounding their version of ethnomethodology,[34] everyday accounts are a 'topic'. They are problematic. They are to be investigated. In the case of ethnomethodology

> ... instead of an ethnography that inventories a setting's distinctive, substantive features, the research vehicle envisioned here is a ***methodography*** ... that searches for the practices through which those substantive features are made observable.[35]

If there is to be a genuinely phenomenological sociology, it must be along these lines, i.e. an attempt to get behind the natural attitude and clarify the grounds on which it is based. Such an endeavour, Zaner tells us,[36] is directed to 'bring out or *make explicit* those structures that remain merely *implicit* and taken for granted, in order to make possible a critical understanding of them and permit their assessment'. It constitutes, Zaner concludes, a 'difficult task'. Gurwitsch agrees that it is difficult. In his view, phenomenological inquiry of this kind

> ... purports nothing less than accounting for the world, its objectivity, and the unquestioned certainty of its existence in subjective terms, or to put it differently, revealing the world as a correlate and product of subjective functions, activities, and operations.[37]

'Accounting for the world'. 'Revealing the world'. This is the paramount aim of mainstream phenomenology. 'For us', says Merleau-Ponty, 'the essential is to know precisely what the being of the world means.'[38] We find this same emphasis in van Manen:

> From a phenomenological point of view, to do research is always to question the way we experience the world, to want to know the world in which we live as human beings. And since to know the world is profoundly to be in the world in a certain way, the act of researching-questioning-theorizing is the intentional act of attaching ourselves to the world, to become more fully part of it, or better, to become the world. Phenomenology calls this inseparable connection to the world the principle of 'intentionality'. In doing research we question the world's very secrets and intimacies which are constitutive of the world, and which bring the world as world into being for us and in us.[39]

This emphasis on the world as intentional *object* is lacking in much of the sociology that claims to be phenomenological. Instead, the emphasis is on the human *subjects* — on their shared ways of perceiving, thinking, acting and interacting. It is accepted that actors socially construct their world and the effort is put into exploring their constructions. A praiseworthy enterprise but, if one rests content with that, it remains an exceedingly subjective enterprise. Turner may have this kind of sociology in mind when he writes that phenomenology 'has frequently become an orgy of subjectivism'.[40] Rather than a questioning of 'the world's very secrets and intimacies which are constitutive of the world', as van Manen puts it, this form of social inquiry is a questioning of the secrets and intimacies of persons.

Schutz, for his part, is concerned with the world — with the phenomenology of the social world and the structure of the lifeworld, as the titles of his works attest. He is clearly not doing what the new phenomenologists do, even if some of them cite him in support of their method.

The new phenomenologists seek to explore in direct fashion the shared perceptions and meanings of others. This does not reflect the Schutzian project, as Natanson underlines:

> Nor is subjectivity to be approached through more sophisticated theories of personal intuition and empathy. Schutz explicitly repudiates the translation of *verstehende Soziologie* into ... a hermeneutics of fellow-feeling which tries to enter directly into the actuality of the Other's lived experience ... The matter does not end there, of course, because my knowledge of the Other in its greatest complexity comes with the typifications and ideal types which form the matrix of social life. The description, analysis, and clarification of that matrix is nothing less than the subject matter of a phenomenology of the social sciences.[41]

Ethnomethodology is concerned with the world too. It wants to understand and explain the coherent, consistent, planful world which we experience. Its exponents may study individuals but they are not on the trail of *experiencing individuals* in order to define and describe their characteristics, not even their social characteristics. As ethnomethodologists, they are after the structure of their *experienced world*. In this, as Gallant and Kleinman point out, they differ from symbolic interactionists.

> In looking for an underlying structure, ethnomethodologists bracket interaction, effectively making actors and their audiences epiph-enomenal. Symbolic interactionists, on the other hand, suspend the assumption of an underlying structure and seek instead to discover social organizational processes.[42]

There were early efforts to maintain the authentic core of phenomenology against the tendency to assimilate phenomenology to the interpretative sociology of the day. Heap and Roth, in an article that appeared originally in 1973, point to approaches which march under the banner of 'phenomenological sociology' but which 'display only a metaphorical understanding of phenomenology as a philosophy and as a set of methods'.[43] Heap and Roth write of the ways in which 'intention', 'reduction', 'phenomenon' and 'essence' are misconstrued.[44] They consider that interpretative social thought in the mode of W I Thomas, Cooley, Mead and Weber can be said to be phenomenological only 'in a loose sense', i.e. as making use of a phenomenological philosophical perspective, even though they may not be aware of doing so.[45] Believing that 'phenomenology, properly understood, can contribute to the sociological enterprise, properly understood', they call for 'systematic and disciplined inquiry into Husserlian phenomenologies and their derivatives (transcendental, psychological, hermeneutical, and existential phenomenologies)'.[46]

Voices like that of Heap and Roth were not listened to. O'Neill regards Heap and Roth's call to orthodoxy as too rigid to be feasible:

They propose to define the adherents of phenomenological sociology in terms of an adequate grasp of four Husserlian concepts: 'intention'; 'reduction'; 'phenomenon'; and 'eidetic structure'. This serves to render phenomenological sociology impossible unless the usage is relaxed, or else honoured by misuse.[47]

For his part, O'Neill is happy to include 'interpretative sociology', carried out in the tradition of W I Thomas, Cooley, Mead and Weber, as one of four types into which the 'actual practice of phenomenological sociology' can be seen to fall.

The diversity of the phenomenological movement has been stressed many times over. Given that diversity, it is difficult to be purist about phenomenology, even if one wants to be. However, it is one thing to reject a rigid orthodoxy in the understanding of phenomenology; it is another thing to reject the notion of a common core in the various phenomenologies and to identify phenomenology with any approach that resembles it in any respect. The price one pays for such unbridled ecumenism is enormous.

For a start, to the extent that phenomenology comes to be identified with other interpretative approaches to social science, it loses its critical character, becoming simply a description of everyday understandings. Here we might heed Schutz's warning that, 'when common-sense assumptions are uncritically admitted into the apparatus of a science, they have a way of taking their revenge'.[48]

For this and other reasons, it is undoubtedly important to distinguish what is phenomenological from what is not phenomenological, even if, as Rehorick suggests, 'it is imperative that risk-taking emissaries continue to straddle the phenomenological and non-phenomenological domains'.[49] Psathas is careful to make the distinction. Of the thinkers to whom Heap and Roth, and then O'Neill, refer, Psathas describes Weber as 'pre-phenomenological', while pointing to the work of Thomas, Cooley and Mead as 'parallel, even converging at times, but more inspiring to the mainstream workers in phenomenology than in the stream themselves'. Contrasting with this is the work of Schutz, which 'represents a genuine immersion in and contribution to phenomenological social science'.[50]

Not that we can look back to Schutz, or the ethnomethodologists, as to some Golden Age where the fruits of phenomenological sociology are waiting to be plucked. To defend them as authentic phenomenologists is not to overlook their shortcomings or the inchoate nature of their initiatives. We may reject the views of those who would deny them the mantle of phenomenology, but that does not mean disregarding the views of their other critics. What of Misgeld who claims that 'phenomenological sociology in its original Schutzian form (and as developed by Berger and Luckmann) cannot be taken to have carried the critique of scientific sociology far enough'?[51] What of Bauman who believes that, while Schutz's project may be effective in critiquing sociology, it cannot do the same for society?

> With all its powerful critical potential aimed at sociology, conceived as the science of unfreedom, the Schutzian alternative refrains from offering a conceptual standpoint from which a critique of social reality (as opposed to the critique of its image) could be launched.[52]

Nor can we simply ignore critics like Harvey who goes further still and states that 'Schutz, Berger and Luckman present not only a theoretically inconsistent form of phenomenology, but one which has lost all its radical foundations'.[53]

Imperfect they are, indeed. Their imperfection notwithstanding, Schutz, the ethnomethodologists and other genuinely phenomenological sociologists point us towards the phenomenological task and the phenomenological goal. The task is laborious, but the goal is rewarding. There is benefit to be gained, for our understanding of society, in getting behind the taken-for-granted meanings, seeing how social reality structures itself in our immediate consciousness and experience of it, and attending 'to what is substantive and nuclear in its givenness'.[54]

This is not to suggest that the phenomenological task is the only sociological task or the phenomenological goal the only sociological goal. Husserl was concerned with 'beginnings' and phenomenology may be viewed as essentially a starting point. A most valuable starting point — an essential starting point, one may wish to argue, and a starting point which is not left behind but accompanies the inquirer at every further step — but by no means the be-all and end-all of social inquiry.

Jeffrey Robinson's 'classroom experiment'[55] in radical literary education may perhaps serve as an exemplar in this respect. Robinson reports on an academic program in which he leads his students in a semester-long focus on a poem by Wordsworth. 'Ode: Intimations of immortality from recollections of early childhood' is a work that has immediate impact on students. Their initial contemplation of this ode is a significant aesthetic experience that issues in a great sense of wonderment.

Robinson, however, is not content to leave it at that. He has known many literature programs which 'satisfy the hunger for order and coherence and the chaste idyll of beauty'. In such programs, he has found, the satisfaction achieved 'rarely bridges the gap between the pastoral play inside the classroom and the life outside of it'. He wants his program to succeed where these other programs fail. He wants it to bridge that gap, for it is a gap that supports students' fantasies about, say, capitalism and capitalism's ability to offer 'a version of the idyll of literary experience'.[56] The assumption 'that the study of literature ought to be "disinterested", or apolitical' was one that Robinson regarded as unchallengeable when he entered the teaching profession. It is one that he has now well and truly jettisoned.

> Literature, as the institution of our education presents it, often becomes — as I will show — an embodiment of a power structure; it retains an authority which tends to force submission to it and its values or codes. Literature in the classroom often perpetuates the association of power and domination with beauty.[57]

So there are compelling issues here for both teachers and students of literature. It is not enough to engage in education from what Robinson terms 'the traditional humanist position'. In such humanist education the great works 'provide a locus of simplicity and coherence and beauty' and 'are a relief, a consolation'. But, left at that, they constitute a 'mutual submission to a form of oppression that distances both teacher and pupil from any form of critical thinking in the name of beauty'. What Robinson wants is 'education for critical consciousness, for which the defining term is *mind*'. This is not 'mind' in Schiller's sense as 'a high form of *play* ... an exhibition and exercise of disinterested freedom and thus a proof of human dignity and the best fruits of a civilized society'. Rather, it is 'mind' as Blake conceives it. '*Mind* for Blake is politically engaged, and so-called disinterested play of mind is a form of tyranny.'[58]

Yes, there are questions here that both teachers and students of literature need to address. In Robinson's case, there are questions that the teacher and the students of Wordsworth's 'Ode' need to address. Within what 'system' has this poem come to be so that it is able to overpower students in the way it does? Under what conditions can they be liberated from the limitations of an aesthetic experience of this kind? Robinson wants students to be aware of these systems and to know these conditions. Wordsworth's 'Ode' stands squarely in the inherited tradition of the dominant class, possessing a reality that differs from that of the literature of the oppressed. Here Robinson comes to invoke Freire-style conscientisation:

> The object of a 'pedagogy of the oppressed' applied to Wordsworth's 'Ode' is to gain critical consciousness of this system or of, as Freire might call it, a set of 'codes' which education is at pains to transmit and which we readily embrace.[59]

So Robinson leads his students in an historical consideration of ode as genre, through a study of Wordsworth's life (and what a political creature he was!), to an examination of how the poem was more than once revised by its author (not simply to make it better but because of certain known pressures on him). William Hazlitt has left us a contemporary critique of this ode and the students come in the end to take full account of this criticism. They may start with the beauty and wonder of a poem but they finish with themselves and their action within their world. '"What for me is the fate of beauty?" was a question asked eventually by many of the students.'[60]

Robinson concludes:

> To bring literature into the realm of politics; to bring fantasy into the realm of effective action; to bring adolescence into its unique exercise of power in the presence of the beautiful, which I hope the years will not diminish, are the goals of this experiment in education.[61]

Such an outcome, says Bogdan,[62] 'is no spectator response, to be sure, but rather the reinfusing of action into literary experience, creating text even as one receives it — mediating verbal and psychic reality as the first step in changing the world.'

What Bogdan finds 'compelling' about this exercise by Robinson is that the initial aesthetic experience is not lost to the students as they explore the political dimension of it all. Indeed, they reach and retain an admirable 'depth of felt poetic understanding'. Here, Bogdan believes, Robinson differs from 'many contemporary literary theorists ... who, in their drive to raise consciousness about the sociological implications of reading literature, feel that they have to construct an enemy out of the aesthetic'.[63]

Can it not be said that in sociology the phenomenologist looks at social realities in much the same way as Robinson's students begin their considerations of Wordsworth's ode? This is the kind of aesthetic experience that Bogdan refers to as *stasis*.

> An intensely personal and private experience, perhaps best manifested as silence, it is usually marked by a recession of cognitive faculties and a near paralysis of linguistic powers.[64]

Phenomenological seeing is *stasis* too. The phenomenologist endeavours to open up to social phenomena, as the objects of immediate experience, to grasp them and be grasped by them, and to describe (with great difficulty) what has come into view. What is thus grasped and expressed forms a broad and firm foundation for what ensues. But a foundation, only — not a total framework, much less the whole fabric. The inquirer will cease to function in phenomenological fashion and may become, say, like one of Robinson's students, a Freirean critic of society. Here (or in whatever other sociological route is followed) attention will need to be given to a whole range of considerations other than what presents itself in immediate experience. One must move from *stasis* to Robinson's 'realm of effective action', 'exercise of power', 'politics', and the rest. But the insights gained from the *stasis* are not rejected. They remain with the inquirer to the end. They serve to guide, to inform, to enhance, to refine, to challenge, to confirm ...

And the initial *stasis* is not the only *stasis*. The inquirer will return to the phenomenological stance time and again. While the sociologist lays the phenomenological mantle aside and moves far afield, what phenomenology offers sociology is not only a beginning rooted in immediate social experience but a methodology that requires a return to that experience at every point along the way. It is both starting point and touchstone.

This is what Merleau-Ponty has in mind when he warns us that, instead of attempting to establish in positivist fashion the things that 'build up the shape of the world', we need to recognise our *experience* of these things 'as the source which stares us in the face and as the ultimate court of appeal in our knowledge of these things'.[65] For Merleau-Ponty, a phenomenological return to experience is 'philosophy' — not philosophy as a particular body of knowledge but philosophy as a vigilance which never lets us forget the origin of all our knowledge. Philosophy of this kind, he insists, is necessary to sociology 'as a constant reminder of its tasks'. Through it 'the sociologist returns to the living sources of his knowledge'.[66]

We can substitute Bogdan's language for that of Merleau-Ponty and say of this kind of sociology that it is no spectator response, 'to be sure'. Rather, in her terms still, it is the reinfusing of action into phenomenological experience, creating social reality even as one receives it — mediating verbal and psychic reality as the first step in changing the world.

Taking that 'first step' demands a specifically phenomenological mode of thinking and investigating on the part of the researcher. It requires a transcending of the natural attitude. Not everyone is ready for it. 'Too many', warns Rehorick, 'remain unaware that there is a "natural attitude" to be transcended.'[67]

NOTES

1 This is surely an 'ethnocentrism' on the part of Anglophone sociologists. What, for example, about Alfred Vierkandt, whose principal works appeared in 1923 and 1926 and who 'was considered the phenomenological sociologist par excellence at that time' (Srubar 1984, p. 179)?

2 'The newer phenomenological approaches are sometimes referred to as 'community-based', 'qualitative', or 'naturalistic' research strategies.' (Murphy 1986, p. 338).

3 Macionis (1991), pp. 155, 168.

4 Benner (1984), p. 218.

5 Diekelmann (1992), p. 73.

6 Mitchell (1977), pp. 115–116.

7 Denzin (1978), p. 99.

8 Psathas (1973), pp. 6–7.

9 Mitchell (1977), p. 117.

10 See Cicourel (1968).

11 Psathas (1973), pp. 14–15.

12 Wolff (1989b), p. 326.

13 Douglas (1974), pp. 113–114.

14 *Ibid.*, p. 190.

15 Natanson (1974), p. 8.

16 Weber (1946), p. 55.
17 Weber (1968), p. 3
18 Lewis (1975), p. 39.
19 Schutz (1967), p. 43.
20 Schutz (1966), p. 82.
21 Schutz (1967), p. 44.
22 *Ibid.*, p. 37.
23 Schutz (1962), p. 42.
24 Schutz (1962), p. 229.
25 Natanson (1977), p. 111.
26 Grossberg (1983).
27 *Ibid.*, p. 100.
28 *Ibid.*, p. 103.
29 Hardin, Power and Sugrue (1986), p. 55.
30 'Thus, ethnomethodology remains neither sociology nor phenomenology.'
     (Islam 1983, p. 149)
31 Bauman (1973), p. 6.
32 Turner (1986), p. 327.
33 *Ibid.*, p. 390.
34 Zimmerman and Pollner (1971), pp. 81–82.
35 *Ibid.*, p. 95.
36 Zaner (1970), p. 82.
37 Gurwitsch (1966), p. 416.
38 Merleau-Ponty (1968), p. 6.
39 van Manen (1990), p. 5.
40 Turner (1986), p. 475.
41 Natanson (1974), p. 47.
42 Gallant and Kleinman (1983), p. 10.
43 Heap and Roth (1978), p. 279.
44 *Ibid.*, pp. 280–284.
45 *Ibid.*, p. 286.
46 *Ibid.*, p. 289.
47 O'Neill (1985), p. 752.
48 Schutz (1967), p. 9.
49 Rehorick (1991), p. 368.
50 Psathas (1973), pp. 2–3.
51 Misgeld (1983), p. 125.
52 Bauman (1976), p. 64.
53 Harvey (1972), p. 106.
54 Natanson (1974), p. 11.
55 See Robinson (1987).
56 *Ibid.*, pp. 4–5.
57 *Ibid.*, p. 14.
58 *Ibid.*, pp. 5–9.
59 *Ibid.*, pp. 13–14.
60 *Ibid.*, *p.* 17.
61 *Ibid.*, p. 185.
62 Bogdan (1990), p. 182.
63 *Ibid.*, p. 181.
64 *Ibid.*, p. 119.
65 Merleau-Ponty (1962), p. 23.
66 Merleau-Ponty (1964b), p. 110.
67 Rehorick (1991), p. 368.

7

Transcending the natural attitude

'It is the task of phenomenology,' says Marton[1] 'to depict the basic structure of our experience of various aspects of reality and to make us conscious of what the world was like before we learned how to see it.'

Attempting to do that calls into question the way in which we see our world. This questioning is very radical questioning, for in the natural attitude, the way in which we make sense of things is taken to be the way things really are. In phenomenology that natural attitude is transcended. What is taken for granted is rendered problematic — not only the obviously taken-for-granted but even the taken-for-granted that has slipped into the background of our awareness. Hardison[2] talks of the way in which a cultural innovation, once it has been assimilated, comes to be taken for granted. This, he says, 'means that, in a sense, it has become obvious and invisible at the same time' and there is need for 'a great deal of contemplating of the invisible in the obvious'. A useful exercise that, but phenomenology goes much further. Phenomenology is not content to contemplate the invisible. As part of what is taken for granted in our understanding of things, the invisible, along with the obvious, is called into question and this means, for purposes of phenomenological inquiry, that it is set aside. It is paid no regard. We must, Natanson tells us, 'step outside the circle of the taken for granted in order to inspect the taken for granted'.[3]

Drawing on Sartre's idea of the nothingness of consciousness, John Wild suggests that in phenomenology 'awareness must in itself be as nothing'. He is not talking of an absolute nothingness. 'Absolute nothingness has no power of any kind.' Instead, he means a return to 'noetic nothingness'. We must be ready to 'examine any question in the light of the evidence alone, apart from all subjective prejudice'. Wild points out that, when our noetic power becomes permanently coloured by some bias, we 'do not understand things as they are in themselves, but only from a certain point of view, as they are mixed with the demands elicited by a certain fixed position'. We need to 'escape from this imprisonment in a world of our own construction'. We need to be 'ready to give one answer or the opposite ... prepared for either being or nothing ... ready to receive being as it is'. As we go back to the things themselves, we 'do not lock them up inside a finite or absolute container of any sort, but rather stretch out our minds to existence'.[4]

Step outside the circle of the taken for granted. Be ready to receive being as it is. Stretch out our minds to existence. How are we to go about doing that? What methods can we use to lay aside accepted meanings, inherited understandings, and prevailing interpretations, so as to grasp, and be grasped by, the phenomena that lie behind them, the objects of experience as they are before they are meant, understood and interpreted in the ways they are? What are the routes available to us as we strive to reach what the phenomena have to offer us from within their very structure? What they have to offer are openings for fresh meaning, scope for deeper under-standing, possibilities of more authentic and more telling interpretation, but how are we to take hold of what they offer?

We might remind ourselves here of Merleau-Ponty's view of things. As he sees it, what appears to us in our perception of the world does not come fitted out with ready-made meaning. The world in itself is very indeterminate. Meaning is not out there in the world simply awaiting our discovery of it. Meaning is unthinkable without the concept of 'mind' — a conscious, experiencing (and embodied) subject. Meanings are not merely encountered and gathered along the way. They are created. They come into being as subject and object relate to each other. They spring from dialogue — mutual interaction — between subject and object.

Indeterminate as it is in its primordiality, the phenomenon still brings with it a certain 'atmosphere' of meaning, says Merleau-Ponty. The phenomenon, we may say, is pregnant with meaning. If that is so, the phenomenologist is midwife. Meaning, Gillan tells us, is 'event'[5] — it 'erupts'[6] — and phenomenology is 'creative act'.[7]

The pain of natural labour

Giving birth, or being creative, is never easy. Phenomenologists, from Husserl onwards, take care to stress the difficulty and painstaking nature of getting back to, and re-encountering, the phenomena of immediate experience. Not everyone is capable of it.

Husserl uses words like 'exacting' and 'laborious' to characterise the phenomenological endeavour:

> That we should set aside all previous habits of thought, see through and break down the mental barriers which these habits have set along

the horizons of our thinking ... — these are hard demands ... To move freely along this new way without ever reverting to the old viewpoints, to learn to see what stands before our eyes, to distinguish, to describe, calls, moreover, for exacting and laborious studies.[8]

'Nothing', says Merleau-Ponty, 'is more difficult to know than precisely *what we see.*'[9] Wild is in agreement: 'To some degree such knowledge is open to us, but only on the condition of long and grueling discipline'.[10]

Writing in the same vein of the 'intuiting' and 'describing' inherent in the phenomenological task, Spiegelberg suggests the need for personal aptitude as well as a readiness to make the effort. Phenomenology, he warns,

... is fully aware that careful intuiting and faithful description are not to be taken for granted and that they require a considerable degree of aptitude, training and conscientious self-criticism'.[11]

While recognising the difficulty and complexity of phenomenological research, we should not allow ourselves the impression that phenomenological seeing is a strange and unnatural pastime. If it is labour, it is natural labour.

In our kind of society we may have moved far from immediate experience of phenomena. We may tend to live our lives isolated — insulated, even — from such experience. That, however, is not a universal condition. Even today there are traditional societies where the culture remains sufficiently intact to preserve a good measure of direct contact with 'original', 'primordial' phenomena, i.e. where people are permitted and called upon to see, hear, feel, smell and touch — and to dwell on — the primary objects of their experience. Their understandings tend to be embodied concretely in myth and ritual, which remain much closer to primary experience than our more rational and abstract explications.

Rollo May has recognised the way in which myth incarnates immediate experience. This recognition has led him to postulate a need for myth and detect a 'cry for myth' in society today. May contrasts the mythical with the empirical, for 'whereas empirical language refers to objective facts, *myth refers to the quintessence of human experience, the meaning and significance of human life*'.[12]

May refers us to Bronislaw Malinowski. Malinowski has much to say about myth:[13]

Myth ..., in its living primitive form, is not merely a story told but a reality lived ...

Studied alive, myth ... is not symbolic, but a direct expression of its subject matter; it is not an explanation in satisfaction of a scientific interest, but a narrative resurrection of a primeval reality, told in satisfaction of deep religious wants, moral cravings, social submissions, assertions, even practical requirements.

By contrasting them with scientific explanation — or, indeed, with any kind of rational explanation — Malinowski is highlighting the way in which myths directly represent experience. The realities they embody do not need explaining, he tells us. For those who have experienced them, the realities are 'only too hauntingly real, too concrete, too easy to comprehend'. Myths are not 'an intellectual reaction upon a puzzle' but simply express this haunting reality, this concreteness, this comprehension, for those who live them out.

They do not want to 'explain', to make 'intelligible' anything which happens in their myths — above all not an abstract idea.

Myth making, then, as an incarnation of primordial experience, may be seen as a phenomenological enterprise. It is interesting that Husserl, in his efforts to illuminate the *Lebenswelt* (for him, the world as experienced immediately by a living subject), looks to what the anthropologist Lucien Lévy-Bruehl has to say about the mythical and magical world of more traditional cultures.[14]

Heidegger, for his part, looks to the early Greeks and to poetry. In Heidegger's developing quest, the thought expressed by the pre-Socratic thinkers reflects primordial experience in a very concrete and direct fashion. As we have noted in an earlier chapter, Heidegger perceives an originality in the thought of the early Greeks ('that which is primally early') which is difficult to find elsewhere and he calls upon us 'to think through still more primally what was primally thought'.[15] We have also noted how Heidegger attributes to poets like Hölderlin a very special role in the manifestation of Being. In many places in his writings, he returns to Hölderlin's claim, '... poetically dwells man upon this earth'.

Poetry's ability to express immediate human experience and remain close to that experience is widely recognised. Its degree of success in doing so, many would want to say, is the very measure of its quality as poetry. To illustrate this, Kaufmann points to Shakespeare. In Kaufmann's judgment, passages in which Shakespeare merely conforms to conventional sentiments tend to be poor poetically because they lack spontaneity and inspiration; on the other hand, 'the speeches that explode convention and give form to Shakespeare's own experience elevate us to an altogether different plane'.[16] From this point of view, it is not difficult to forge a close link between poetry and phenomenology. Phenomenologists too seek to explode conventional ways of seeing the world and give form to their actual experience of it.

Heidegger expressly forges such a link. He brings together 'thinking' (*Denken* — the word which, as we have already seen, emerges in Heidegger's vocabulary as the word 'phenomenology' recedes) and 'poetry'. 'Poetry and thought are not the same thing', he says. Nevertheless, at their best, both are 'essentially superior to the spirit that prevails in all mere science'.

By virtue of this superiority the poet always speaks as if the essent [that which has being] were being expressed and invoked for the first time. Poetry, like the thinking of the philosopher, has always so much world space to spare that in it each thing — a tree, a mountain, a house, the cry of a bird — loses all indifference and commonplaceness.[17]

'So', writes van Manen, drawing on Merleau-Ponty rather than Heidegger, 'phenomenology, not unlike poetry, is a poetizing project; it tries an incantative, evocative speaking, a primal telling, wherein we aim to involve the voice in an original singing of the world.'[18]

In this relationship between phenomenology and poetry, the Russian Formalists have yet another dimension to offer us. In this school of literary criticism, poetry came to be seen as doing violence to language and, through the deformity it causes in language, bringing about *ostranenie*, a 'making strange'. *Ostranenie* is an attempt to 'counteract the process of habituation encouraged by routine everyday modes of perception'.[19] It is 'the making strange of reality in order to create it anew'.[20] This is precisely what phenomenology strives to do through the 'reduction' it effects by way of bracketing or *epoché*.

> We very readily cease to 'see' the world we live in, and become very anaesthetized to its distinctive features. The aim of poetry is to reverse that process, to *defamiliarize* that with which we are overly familiar, to 'creatively deform' the usual, the normal, and so to inculcate a new, childlike, non-jaded vision in us. The poet thus aims to disrupt 'stock responses' and to generate a heightened awareness: to restructure our ordinary perception of 'reality', so that we may end by *seeing* the world instead of numbly recognizing it; or at least so that we end by designing a 'new' reality to replace the (no less fictional) one which we have inherited and become accustomed to.[21]

Here Terence Hawkes is expounding the insights of Russian Formalist Viktor Shklovsky, but the passage would still make complete sense if one were to substitute 'phenomenology' for 'poetry' and 'phenomenologist' for 'poet'.

Nor need we limit the comparison to poetry. All the arts have an affinity to phenomenology. Merleau-Ponty points not only to Valéry but to Balzac, Proust and Cézanne and states that phenomenology shares with their works 'the same kind of attentiveness and wonder, the same demand for awareness, the same will to seize the meaning of the world or of history as that meaning comes into being'.[22]

Anthropologist Clifford Geertz speaks in this vein of the 'aesthetic attitude'. It involves, he tells us, a suspension of naive realism and practical interest.

> Instead of questioning the credentials of everyday experience, that experience is merely ignored in favor of an eager dwelling upon

appearances, an engrossment in surfaces, an absorption in things, as we say, 'in themselves'.[23]

Philosopher Susanne Langer makes the same point. Art involves 'disengagement from belief — the contemplation of sensory qualities without their usual meanings'.[24] The content of artistic forms, Langer insists, is 'pure appearance', which makes these forms 'more freely and wholly apparent than they could be if they were exemplified in a context of real circumstance and anxious interest'.[25]

In the Romantic tradition, literary educationalist Jeffrey Robinson points out, beauty is the distinguishing element of art and it summons us, not to reason, but to wonder:

> The experience of beauty requires the suspension of the critical faculty, the transcendence of a comprehending response to the world, the suppression of the fantasy life except for idyllic fantasies ... Mind, in its analytical, critical capacity, acting only as a fallen instrument of ordering life in a fallen world, ceases to act in the presence of beauty and, as Keats says, ends in speculation or wonderment. [26]

We cannot just continue in such wonderment. If, through this kind of aesthetic experience, our mind ceases to act in its habitual fashion, it begins at once to work again, albeit in a different way. We may have left taken-for-granted understandings behind, but their place comes to be occupied by new or at least renewed understandings. It is not surprising that this should happen. Indeed, it is important that it happen. In some perspectives, it is essential that it happen. Feminist writer Adrienne Rich[27] addresses this necessity. In pointing up the kind of oppression that women suffer under patriarchy, she directs them to the literature they have inherited. Rich writes of 'the visible effects on women's lives of seeing, hearing our wordless or negated experience affirmed and pursued further in language'. Language has trapped women as well as liberated them. The very act of naming has been until now the prerogative of males. What Rich calls for is 're-vision' — a radical feminist critique of literature which will use literature as a clue to how women have been living and how women can 'begin to see and name — and therefore live — afresh'. 'We need', says Rich, to know the writing of the past, and know it differently than we have ever known it; not to pass on a tradition but to break its hold on us.'

Not to pass on a tradition but to break its hold on us ...
Causing things to lose all indifference and commonplaceness ...
Exploding convention and giving form to experience ...
A narrative resurrection of primeval reality ...
An absorption in things in themselves ...
The contemplation of sensory qualities without their usual meanings ...
A suspension of the critical faculty ...

The mind ceasing to act and ending in wonderment ...
Seeing the world instead of numbly recognising it ...
Speaking as if the object were being expressed and invoked for the
first time ...
To see and name — and therefore live — afresh ...

The parallel between this litany and the task with which phenomenology presents us needs no underlining. Suggesting that we get in touch with the phenomena that present themselves in our immediate experience is not such an outlandish proposal after all. Phenomenological description may stem from formal endeavours on the part of the phenomenologist, but it has genuine affinity to the concrete imagery found in the myths and rituals of more traditional cultures, the thought patterns of early civilisations, and the poetry and other art forms of our own. 'The attempt to recover a fresh perception of existence, one unprejudiced by acculturation, is difficult', says Sadler,[28] 'but it is neither impossible nor fantastic.'

Indeed, there are moments in the lives of every one of us when we go 'back to the things themselves' in spontaneous fashion. These are times — traumatic, turbulent, or at least dislocating, times — when, for one reason or another, our usual way of making sense of things no longer works and we are forced to look at our situation anew.[29] In such moments we may feel we are seeing things for the very first time. Zorba the Greek, presented by Kazantzakis as one who 'lived the earth, water, the animals and God, without the distorting intervention of reason', had such moments:

'What is that?' he asked stupefied. 'That miracle over there, boss, that moving blue, what do they call it? Sea? And what's that wearing a flowered green apron? Earth? Who was the artist who did it? It's the first time I've seen that, boss, I swear!'[30]

If Zorba's reaction seems a long way from talk of phenomenological reduction, we might recall the phrase used by Husserl's assistant, Eugen Fink. It is a phrase which Merleau-Ponty thinks may well be the best formulation of the phenomenological reduction.[31] Spiegelberg translates it as 'shock of amazement at the fact of the world'. What Fink had in mind, Spiegelberg explains, is 'a stunned wonderment to which he assigned the function of converting the trivial into what is worth questioning'.[32]

Little children are very capable of this shock of amazement, this stunned wonderment, to which Fink and Spiegelberg refer. We tend to lose our ready sense of wonder as we develop. Schachtel[33] describes how our perception comes to be organised differently as we move from childhood into adulthood. Where the child's perception remains close to the immediate situation ('the actual riches, spontaneity, freshness of childhood experience'), the adult's becomes distanced from it. Worse, the living perception comes to be replaced by the prevailing understanding of its object.

In the course of later childhood, adolescence, and adult life, perception and experience themselves develop increasingly into the rubber stamps of conventional clichés. The capacity to see and feel what is there gives way to the tendency to see and feel what one expects to see and feel, which, in turn, is what one is expected to see and feel because everybody else does.[34]

Phenomenology is about redeveloping this 'capacity to see and feel what is there'. It is an attempt to regain a childlike openness in our encounter with the world.

The conclusion is clear. What people in more traditional cultures do in the course of their day-to-day involvements and express in myth and ritual, what poets and other aesthetes do in their artistic labours, what we have done as children in very spontaneous fashion and even now do perforce in special moments of our lives — this is what phenomenology calls upon us to do in deliberate, self-conscious, painstaking fashion.

If we accept the invitation, the question posed at the start of this chapter emerges for us again and with urgency. In what way — by what steps — are we to 'do' phenomenology?

Let's do it!

Here, then, is a stepwise method for phenomenological research that uses the phenomenon of nursing as an example.

Step 1

Determine as precisely as possible what phenomenon we are focusing on. *We put the question: what counts as nursing?*

Step 2

Consider the phenomenon precisely as phenomenon.
We take nursing purely as phenomenon, i.e. as it appears in our experience of it, and ask ourselves: what is nursing like? ... what does nursing strike us as being?
This requires that we:

* lay aside, as far as we can, all ideas, judgments, feelings, assumptions, connotations and associations that normally come into view for us when we think of this phenomenon
  We disregard, as far as we can, all that we know about nursing's origins and history, all the expositions of nursing we have read, all the understandings of nursing we have come to accept, everything we have come to associate with

nursing. We try to look on nursing as if it were the first time we have encountered it.

- open ourselves to the phenomenon as the object of our immediate experience
We focus on nursing as a human phenomenon in a sustained and penetrating, but not discursive, fashion.

Step 3

Describe what has come into view for us.
We say what nursing appears to be in our immediate experience of it (taking care to describe nursing and not ourselves).

Step 4

Ensure the phenomenological character of this description.
We look closely at our allegedly phenomenological description and ask whether what we are saying of nursing does genuinely stem from our experience of it as a human phenomenon. Or does it spring, rather, from some other source? … from our awareness of nursing's origin and history? … from theories elaborated about the meaning and purpose of nursing? … from associations with nursing which we learned to make in the course of our socialisation? … from ??? If what we are attributing to nursing comes from anything other than immediate experience of nursing, we jettison it.

Step 5

Determine the essence of the phenomenon, i.e. the element or elements in the phenomenon as phenomenon that make it precisely what it is.
We ask: what is it, in our immediate experience of nursing, that makes nursing nursing? If nursing has appeared to us as 'this' and as 'that', how essential are 'this' and 'that'? Would it still be nursing if 'this' and 'that' were not there?

We need to consider these steps in more detail.

Having carefully determined the phenomenon we wish to focus on and delineate (Step 1), we make every effort to view that phenomenon purely as phenomenon, i.e. as it presents itself to us in our very experience of it. This is Step 2 and it has both a negative and a positive dimension. The negative is to serve the positive. If we 'lay aside', 'hold in abeyance', 'suspend' and the like, it is in order to 'open ourselves to', 'surrender to', 'allow ourselves to be grasped by', and the like.

Let us address the negative side of things first. It is often called 'bracketing'.

Bracketing

To say that phenomenological seeing is not a strange or unnatural activity is to say the same of bracketing in particular. We are always selective in our perception of situations, focusing on certain aspects and ignoring others. We have the ability to prescind from certain features of the object of our attention. In other words, we can just leave them out of consideration for the time being. This can be seen at times to result in a one-sided, distorted understanding or presentation but, as it happens, we need to be selective in order to proceed at all. Without such selectivity, we would be ever confronted and overwhelmed by William James' 'blooming, buzzing confusion'.

Scientists can serve as an example here. Scientists have to bracket out all kinds of features attaching to the objects of their study in order to focus on what they want to focus on. Water will have all kinds of association for chemists. Steam will have another cluster of associations. Ice would have yet another. But, whether it is ice, steam or liquid water chemists are dealing with, they have to lay aside all associations of that kind and consider the object of their attention simply as H_2O.

So bracketing in itself is a normal enough activity. That, as has already been stressed, is not to say that it is easy. To lay aside all our previous thinking and feeling about a phenomenon and try to look at it with fresh eyes takes discipline and persistence. Given such discipline and persistence, however, there would seem to be no inherent reason why the exercise should not be successful, especially since Step 4 is still to come and will test the phenomenological character of what we say has appeared for us.

Opening ourselves to immediate experience

The positive side of Step 2 is our opening of ourselves to the phenomenon itself to the exclusion of all else that relates to it.

As mentioned earlier, the notion that Kurt Wolff uses to describe this exercise is that of *surrender*. We surrender. We yield. We become passive before the phenomenon and allow it to grasp us and impress itself upon us. This, as Wolff has not been slow to point out, stands in stark contrast to the mode of proceeding that characterises any culture shaped by Western science and technology. That is a mode of domination, control and manipulation. Here, in phenomenological inquiry, we have no desire to dominate or control or manipulate.[35] We are content to remain open and passive, allowing the phenomenon to give itself to us as it is.

Heidegger uses the word *Gelassenheit* to describe this kind of openness and passivity. *Gelassenheit* is often translated simply as 'serenity', but it really means a 'releasedness', a 'letting go and letting be'. It is a word prominent in the vocabulary of Meister Eckhart and the Rhineland mystics generally. Its use by Heidegger marks a dramatic shift from the voluntarism of his earlier talk about resoluteness, struggle and doing violence to texts. Now the emphasis is on simply opening ourselves and awaiting the advent of Being. So, in our phenomenological endeavours, we can draw guidance from Heidegger's language here. We need to release ourselves from the whole constellation of concepts and affectivity with which we surround the phenomenon in question. We need to let these go and let the phenomenon be.

Take trees as an example. In infancy and childhood we learned the meaning of trees from the culture in which we were reared. It was given a name for us and, along with the name, a host of meanings and associations. What those meanings and association are depends on the kind of culture or sub-culture we were raised in. For us as adults, if we were reared in a slum neighbourhood with no trees, trees probably have little significance at all. If the setting of our childhood was a logging town, trees would have much meaning as the origin of timber and a source of livelihood. They are best seen, we might want to say, after they have come to maturity and before they become 'over-mature'. If we grew up in an artists' colony where our role models sought to capture the beauty of trees in what they painted and sculpted, it is perhaps the aesthetic aspect of trees that predominates for us. For us, then, they are best seen in the full light of day as the sun brightens the rugged brownness of the trunks and brings a sparkle to the green leaves. If we came to adulthood in an animist community in which spirit life is perceived in trees as in everything else that surrounds us, trees hold a mystical significance for us. They are at their best as the darkness gathers about them each evening and eerie figures emerge from the shadows of their branches and begin to dance among them.

Whatever their provenance, it is these meanings imparted by our culture that come to the fore when we see trees. Our encounter with trees is little more than an occasion for these meanings to flood in upon us. The meanings do not spring from our engagement with these trees or those trees. We bring these meanings ready-made to whatever trees we happen to observe. Or, as Ortega y Gasset would prefer to put it, these meanings are masks worn by trees in our day-to-day experience of them. They are screens that hide trees from us. If we wish to see trees themselves and not merely things-that-have-to-do-with-trees, we have to remove the masks and penetrate the screens.

Thus, whatever their provenance, the meanings we have inherited or borrowed are confining and obstructive: they tend to block out the experience of trees we might have here and now. Whether we are children of slumdwellers, loggers, artists or animists, there are rewards to be found in surrendering ourselves to trees — not trees as peripheral objects that are absent from our childhood memories, not trees as potential sawlogs and pulpwood, not trees as suitable objects to paint and sculpt, not trees as the habitat of otherworldly beings, but simply *trees presenting themselves to us here and now*.

This notion of surrender is a 'dynamic' concept. A more visual notion is that of *contemplation*. Contemplation is the antithesis of discursive reasoning. In discursive reasoning, the mind is active. In contemplation, the mind is passive and receptive. When we contemplate a tree, we do not actively think about it, analyse it, assess it, or attribute properties to it. In contemplating a tree, we simply have the tree before our eyes, at least our mind's eye, and allow it to give itself to our eyes and to our mind. Being contemplative conjures up the notion of being quiet, inactive, at rest. As a number of phenomenological writers have made a point of saying, phenomenology begins in silence. Husserl talks of 'meditating'. 'Here', Scheler reminds us, 'one talks a little less, remains more silent, and sees more.'[36]

This element of passivity and receptivity is inherent in the very notion of *listening*. By its nature, the idea of listening lends itself to characterising the phenomenological endeavour. In phenomenological inquiry, we listen to the phenomena, simply waiting to hear what they have to say to us.

In the notion of listening, as in the notion of contemplation, there is a contrast with discursive reasoning. Heidegger, who sets great store by listening, declares that 'hearing constitutes the primary and authentic way in which *Dasein* is open to its ownmost potentiality for being'[37] and invites us to lay reasoning aside and just listen. Reasoning is to be laid aside, not thought. Our thinking must be permitted to hear the cry that is there to be heard.

> And the ear of our thinking, does it still not hear the cry? It will refuse to hear it so long as it does not begin to think. Thinking begins only when we have come to know that reason, glorified for centuries, is the most stiff-necked adversary of thought.[38]

According to Levin, what Heidegger is calling upon us to do is to 'practise a thinking hearing: a thinking which listens, a listening that is thoughtful'. It is this kind of listening and this kind of thinking that Levin himself posits in contradistinction to 'reason':

> The way of thinking that will be open to an experience with Being, as speculative 'reason' never has been, needs to be a way of thinking deeply intertwined with an ontologically developed listening.[39]

Gabriel Marcel uses the analogy of listening also. He links it to music. For Marcel, experience is mystery. It is an error, he tells us, 'to take experience for granted and to ignore its mystery'.[40] How, then, are we to explore the mystery of experience? Obviously not by reasoning discursively and logically about it, for Marcel is quick to point up the contrast between his 'phenomenological description' and any kind of 'logical schema'.[41]

Far from reasoning about experience, we are simply to listen to it — as musicians might listen to voices joined with them in producing a symphony. As phenomenologists, we listen to what is for us a grand symphony of being.[42]

In phenomenological inquiry, then, we set reasoning aside. We do not call on preconceived or prevailing notions and beliefs to explain what we are experiencing. We let the phenomenon speak for itself. In this vein, the renowned phenomenologist Emmanuel Levinas says of the equally renowned phenomenologist Martin Buber that the latter's descriptions are truly phenomenological because 'they are all based on the concrete reality of perception and do not require any appeal to abstract principle for their justification'.[43] No, in phenomenology, instead of reasoning about the phenomenon, we simply open ourselves to the phenomenon. We surrender to it. We contemplate it. We listen to it.

What is giving itself to us in this moment?
What is presenting itself to our gaze?
What is this phenomenon saying to us?
What does this phenomenon strike us as being?
These are the phenomenological questions.

Seeing the Grand Canyon

In a celebrated essay,[44] Walker Percy writes about 'seeing' the Grand Canyon. His perceptive analysis illustrates very well what we mean when we talk of opening ourselves to the phenomenon and allowing the phenomenon to give itself to us as it is.

'Garcia López de Cárdenas,' Percy reminds us, 'discovered the Grand Canyon and was amazed at the sight.' One can well understand the amazement. This Spanish explorer was utterly unprepared for what he was now seeing stretched before him. There had been no warning that he might come upon such a scene. There were no expectations. There could be no preconceptions. One can imagine him standing there, open-mouthed, full of wonderment, just allowing the vista to impress itself upon him.

For a long time now the area has been set aside as a national park and a thriving tourist industry has sprung up about it. Week by week, thousands of visitors come to the Grand Canyon seeking to experience what de Cárdenas experienced. But they never do.

Why is it almost impossible to gaze directly at the Grand Canyon under these circumstances and see it for what it is — as one picks up a strange object from one's back yard and gazes directly at it? It is almost impossible because the Grand Canyon, the thing as it is, has been appropriated by the symbolic complex which has already been formed in the sightseer's mind. Seeing the canyon under approved circumstances is seeing the symbolic complex head on. The thing is no

163

longer the thing as it confronted the Spaniard; it is rather that which has already been formulated — by picture postcard, geography book, tourist folders, and the words *Grand Canyon*. As a result of this preformulation, the source of the sightseer's pleasure undergoes a shift. Where the wonder and delight of the Spaniard arose from his penetration of the thing itself, from progressive discovery of depths, patterns, colors, shadows, etc., now the sightseer measures his satisfaction *by the degree to which the canyon conforms to the preformed complex.*[45]

Is it possible for the sightseer to regain de Cárdenas' experience of the Grand Canyon? Percy believes there are several ways of doing so.

For one thing, it may just happen. In a time of national disaster, for instance. The Bright Angel Lodge has been turned into a convalescent home. Someone wounded is brought in. That person regains consciousness and there, outside the window, is the canyon. The patient does not know what it is. Like the Spanish explorer, this wounded person brings no expectations or 'symbolic complex' to the event. The canyon simply hits the eyes and the mind with full force.

Percy also offers what he sees as the 'most extreme case of access by privilege conferred by disaster'. In Huxleyan mode, he conjures up the adventures of a surviving remnant after the great wars of the twentieth century. A group from Australia lands in California, heads east, and comes upon the ruins of the Bright Angel Lodge. 'The trails are grown over, the guard rails fallen away, the dime telescope at Battleship Point rusted.' But the canyon is there. And it is exposed at last — exposed, ironically, by the falling away of the very facilities designed to help the sightseer to see it.

But it need not just happen, this recovery of the de Cárdenas experience. One may deliberately plan to have such an experience. One may decide to follow the Inside Track.

The tourist leaves the tour, camps in the back country. He arises before dawn and approaches the South Rim through a wild terrain where there are no trails and no railed-in lookout points. In other words, he sees the canyon by avoiding all the facilities for seeing the canyon.[46]

The concordance of this account with the description of phenomenological inquiry should be obvious. Each of us has been endowed by our respective culture with 'facilities for seeing' — that system of significant symbols which allows us to communicate and indeed to think. Our birth not merely introduces us to a physical world but ushers us into a pre-constituted, pre-formulated world of meanings. We should be grateful for that. It is what makes us human. Nevertheless, while our culture enables us to experience in human fashion, it also constructs the experience for us in no uncertain manner. It may function as a set of lenses that brings things into view for us, things we would not otherwise see at all, but in doing so it shapes for us what we see. And, let us remember, seeing things 'this' way precludes our seeing things 'that' way. Indeed, seeing things 'this' way precludes our seeing things in their immediacy and so shuts us off from the myriad ways in which they might perhaps be construed. The symbolic complex, as we have seen, is limiting as well as liberating. It is at once boon and burden.

Can we lay that burden aside? Not entirely, for as humans we cannot function without it. We may grant, with Gendlin, 'that phenomenological givens first appear as given, as just *this* given, only after linguistic explication and its assumptions and schemes'.[47] But we can ease the burden. We can stretch the limits. In regard to *this* phenomenon, we can lay aside what we have learnt and bring to our construing of it — just as sightseers may lay aside all that they know or expect or have been led to believe of the Grand Canyon.

What they cannot lay aside is their history. The sightseers remain the persons that they are. As they contemplate the Grand Canyon, the tourist from Buenos Aires and the tourist from Birmingham bring their cultural and individual histories to the task. Because that is so, they will have different experiences of the Grand Canyon. They will make different sense of it. Yet, if they have followed Percy's Inside Track, what presents itself to each of them to be made sense of will be much the same, and the sense they make of it, each in his or her own way, will have an authenticity. It will be *their* sense — not a sense constructed for them by travel brochures or guide books (or, for that matter, by geology textbooks).

Sometimes the laying aside is done for us. Like Percy's wounded patient or surviving remnant, we may find ourselves at times without the benefit of the pre-formulated meanings. As we have already noted, these tend to be times of disruption and trauma. We are dislocated. Our everyday meanings no longer work for us. We are forced to look at things with fresh eyes — as if it were the first time we have ever looked at them — and to make sense of them all over again. These are phenomenological moments, indeed.

Such instances apart, we are left to our own devices. If we want phenomenological moments, we have to create them for ourselves. We have to look to the phenomena alone ('Back to the things themselves!') in very deliberate and painstaking fashion, laying aside all else. The preconceptions, meanings, assumptions, expectations and associations relating to the phenomenon — all these have to go, insofar as they contribute to the sense we make of it. We are taking the Inside Track. We shun the beaten path, with its guide rails, its lookout points and its literature. We walk straight past the interpretation centres with their video sessions and their displays. We seek to be confronted by nothing but the canyon itself in its primordial reality.

No easy task, to be sure. And no doubt, in the end, we must rest content with less than total success. Yet the Inside Track is still worth taking. It may not offer a de Cárdenas experience in its pristine fullness. Yet who would deny that it has so much more to offer — something inestimably richer and more genuine — than anything captured in postcard images, however glossy, or the words of a guide book, however well written?

The question of language

Step 3 requires that we describe what has come into view for us.

This is far more problematic than it sounds. Gendlin has already reminded us that we cannot come to understand what presents itself in our immediate experience, let alone describe it, without the help of language with all 'its assumptions and schemes'. Kullman and Taylor are right in pointing out that 'what is describable or described in language whose logic is predicative, is no longer correctly described as the pre-predicative'.[48]

What this means is that, try as we may to get back to the pre-reflective, to the primordial, to the phenomenal object itself, we find in the end that we cannot take hold of it. It inevitably eludes our grasp. We discover that we can understand it and describe it only in and through thought patterns deriving from our culture and embedded therefore in our language. For that reason, phenomenology is inescapably a hermeneutics. Our phenomenological descriptions cannot but be interpretations and constructions. Using language, Merleau-Ponty tells us, means 'the subject's taking up a position in the world of his meanings'.[49]

From the phenomenological point of view, the best we can do is to minimise the influence wielded by our culturally derived set of meanings via the language we use. We can very deliberately look to putting language at the service of phenomenological description and not the other way round. In short, we try hard to ensure that our attempts to describe do not become a mere imposition of social meaning already to hand.

This has very real implications for our use of language and has long been recognised as an issue within phenomenology. In his Introduction to Being and Time[50] Heidegger apologises for the 'awkwardness and "inelegance" of expression' in the pages that follow. If, he tells his readers, we are not merely talking about entities but grasping entities 'in their Being', we discover that we lack most of the words we need for the task and, above all, we lack the grammar. As it happens, the reason Heidegger comes to give for failing to complete Being and Time is that he lacks the language to do so. What he goes on to do, of course, is to experiment boldly with language. He is famous for his neologisms, so frustrating for some readers, so fascinating for others. Noting that the invention of new words is a frequent symptom in schizophrenia, phenomenological psychotherapist Viktor Frankl recounts how he once asked an audience to consider two passages, one cited from Heidegger and the other from a schizophrenic patient. He invited the members of his audience to assign

166

each of the passages to its respective author. The majority, Frankl reports, 'mistook the words of one of the greatest philosophers of all times for the words of the severely disturbed patient, and vice versa'.

> However, this does not speak against Heidegger but rather against man's capacity to verbalize through the medium of everyday words the experience of a world hitherto unknown, either the world of a new philosophy or that in which a schizophrenic patient is doomed to live. The common denominator is not the expression of a psychotic crisis but rather a crisis of semantic expression.[51]

Frankl is right. When we try to describe what presents itself to us in our very experience of it, we are lost for words. In the face of what Frankl terms 'a world hitherto unknown', our everyday vocabulary proves inadequate and distorting and we are forced to be as resourceful and inventive as we can. 'Creative writing' takes on new meaning, for here we are not looking for literary merit of any kind. Our task is not that of creating new expressions or new forms of writing for their own sake. Our task is simply that of articulating what stands before us — the object of our experience confronting us in its stark immediacy and therefore appearing to us, in Merleau-Ponty's terms, as strange and paradoxical.

Merleau-Ponty himself has to struggle with language. For a start, we find him taking standard terms and infusing new meaning into them. For example, in Merleau-Ponty's hands, the word *perception* becomes 'a nascent logos'; it is 'our presence at the moment when things, truths, values are constituted for us'. This, as Ihde points out,[52] is to impose on the word a load it is not usually asked to bear. However, Merleau-Ponty does much more than clothe common words in new usages. We find him coining new terms (like 'lived body') and drawing on diverse contexts to provide words and phrases ('flesh', 'chiasm', 'perceptual faith') and especially metaphors ('gestural meaning', 'singing the world'). This, in the end, is what Ihde describes as 'wild language'. Much more than a mere transformation of words and phrases, it is 'the initiation of a radical discourse'.

If Merleau-Ponty is forced to wrestle with language, it has to be said that he well and truly wins out. John O'Neill writes of the 'solicitation of Merleau-Ponty's thought and language'.

> Merleau-Ponty's fascination with language and symbols, the wonder of art and vision, the ambivalence of history and action, is a fascination with the origin of things, nature and man. Thus his own language seems to caress the contours of things; often his thoughts achieve a tactile quality which results in a cathexis of thought and being, a logos, in which the word becomes flesh. In short, there is a magic in Merleau-Ponty's language which makes being sensible to us and in turn opens us to its peculiar solicitation.[53]

To the extent that we succeed in getting behind inherited and prevailing understandings and identifying the objects to which they relate, we too will find ourselves struggling with language as we attempt to describe what we see. What do we need, then? 'Wild language', as Ihde says? 'Evocative, incantative speaking ... not unlike poetry', as van Manen would have it? If that seems to be asking too much, let us at least recognise the difficulties we face in describing our phenomena and the need to be as resourceful and skilful as we can in our use of language for that purpose.[54]

And, yes, let us freely acknowledge that, no matter how linguistically creative we turn out to be, our phenomenological seeing will still not issue in a presuppositionless description of immediate experience. For all our investigation of it, Marcel tells us, the mystery of being remains mystery and cannot be converted into the content of thought. We cannot really describe that mystery; we can only allude to it as poets and musicians do.[55] No, what we arrive at is not pure description of pure phenomena. It is reinterpretation, reconstruction, a remaking of sense. A much more modest outcome but, imperfect as it inevitably will be, it is precisely what we set out to achieve.

Are we there?

Being unable to describe fully and faithfully what appears to us in our immediate experience is one thing. Substituting everyday understandings for that immediate experience is another. In our phenomenological endeavours, we will not simply assume that we have successfully reached behind everyday meanings and encountered the 'things themselves'. When we have described what appears to us in our experience of it, the next task (Step 4) is to ask ourselves seriously whether what we describe originates solely in our experience or whether it has come from some other source. Kaelin says of the early phenomenologist Roman Ingarden that he is 'true to his method in not importing anything to the work except what he finds in an experience of it'.[56] That is the litmus test we apply to our own work. Have we 'imported' anything to our description of the phenomenon? Is there anything in that description that has not stemmed authentically from our experience of it?

The next step (Step 5) tests whether what we are describing is of the essence. Is what we are describing that which makes the phenomenon the phenomenon that it is? Would it be this phenomenon if what we are describing were not there? Is what we are describing really characteristic of the phenomenon as precisely *this* phenomenon, distinguishing it from other, perhaps similar, phenomena?

Suppose we were to conclude from our experience of nursing that it presents itself to us as a mutual interpersonal relationship characterised by trust on the part of the client and commitment on the part of the nurse.

In Step 5 we ask whether this is truly of the essence of nursing. For a start, we would surely find it difficult to see such a relationship as specifically characteristic of nursing. It hardly distinguishes nursing from many other professional health services. But the question we need to ask before all else is this: Can there be nursing *without* a mutual interpersonal relationship of this kind? Some possible instances immediately leap to mind. What of the nursing experienced in, say, casualty services, intensive care units and operating theatres? At least part of such nursing is done in circumstances which clearly preclude the development of any such relationship. We may well have decided in Step 1 that nursing in Casualty, Intensive Care and Theatre counts as nursing. Moreover, we may be able to cite further examples where, for reasons other than the setting, no such relationship has developed but nursing is still experienced as nursing. If so, we would be led to conclude that a mutual interpersonal relationship of this kind is not of the essence of nursing.

So we do all that. And, having done all that, how can we be sure that we have captured the essence of the phenomenon as it gives itself to us in experience? Obviously, given the epistemological underpinnings of the phenomenological method, there will be no objective criterion for determining that, if by 'objective' is meant anything like what positivists mean by it. Still, there is a criterion we can point to. It consists in the very 'Aha!' we give when we finally describe what is of the essence. We have a sense that, at last, the description fits. We feel gripped by the phenomenon understood in the way we are describing it. Natanson writes of 'an irreducible presentation, an experiential requiredness which seizes the individual and commands his perceptual assent'. Natanson[57] uses the example of someone 'leaving a tenement room to rush into the swirl and hubbub of a fast-paced and heavily thronged street'. Suddenly, one is *in* the street, pushing and being pushed, caught in the city's reckless din. The 'directly experienced' here, Natanson concludes, is *what is so.*

In short, we describe the phenomenon in the way we do because we feel compelled to understand the phenomenon in the way we do.

Not that we should take the word 'compelled' too absolutely. We are not looking to resurrect Husserl's 'apodicticity'. It is possible, in fact, to have a series of 'ahas' about a single phenomenon and one may come to replace another. As Gendlin points out,[58] this does not make the explication arbitrary. Those descriptions remain genuinely phenomenological which render explicit what hitherto has remained implicit, i.e. our 'pre-ontological being-in-the-world'. The phenomenological description 'draws a response from the implicit' and it is in that response we find the criterion we are looking for. There are other descriptions that will fail to draw such a response. Indeed, Gendlin says, in the face of many descriptions, 'I only feel that vague tired feeling which has not budged with all my good explanations.' But there comes a moment when a response *is* drawn from the implicit. There comes a time when the vague tired feeling well and truly budges. There comes a description which does evoke something in the inquirer and it does so in vital and compelling fashion. That is the description we are seeking and we feel confident in espousing it.

It is like being struck by lightning. Hyperbole? Well, if that seems to be going too far, we can console ourselves that we are not the first to do so. A 'lightning model' is invoked in expositions of literary critical theory.[59] Godzich, for one, explores this analogy very incisively.[60]

Lightning is capricious. It strikes where it will. Disconcerting, but we should make the most of it when it does. Heidegger offers the same injunction by way of a different analogy: he talks repeatedly of 'paths' and 'byways' and 'timber tracks' to indicate that, as we travel on, we often just happen upon 'clearings' where Being is lit up for us. So, in phenomenological inquiry we need to be on the alert for phenomenological moments. We may be reading poetry or other forms of literature, or gazing at art forms of one kind or another, and we recognise with a start that this is the real thing: not the recounting or portrayal of traditional or commonly held understandings but a genuine expression by the author or artist of what is immediately and personally experienced. Or we are engaged in casual conversation and suddenly we strike paydirt in mere *obiter dicta* — passing comments, throw-away lines even — where perhaps assiduous formal interviewing has failed to yield what we are after. In such moments we have the sense that what we are reading or seeing or hearing springs from experience itself and from no other source. We recognise in it Merleau-Ponty's 'natal bonding' of the perceiver with the perceived. It strikes us forcibly that what is being described to us is the phenomenon, as Moustakas puts it, 'in its absolutely native state'. Yes, we value such moments and do not want them to pass us by unexploited.

Yet, as social inquirers, we cannot just wait for such moments to occur. We cannot be content simply to be on the lookout for lightning strikes. Lightning is unpredictable. The challenge, Godzich points out, is to ensure, through disciplined training of perception, not only 'that lightning does strike' but 'that it strike repeatedly, at will, in the same place and with the same intensity'. The 'Aha!' we have been talking about is drawn from us spontaneously at times, but in phenomenological inquiry we look for it in deliberate and methodical fashion.

Working with others

Phenomenological research of the kind proposed here is clearly a first-person exercise. To disregard prior assumptions and understandings and look hard at what presents itself primordially in experience is obviously something one must do for oneself in relation to one's personal experience.

It is not possible to take someone else's account of experience and somehow strip away the everyday interpretations and reach the phenomena as they give themselves to that person. People must do that for themselves.[61]

This sounds as if, to work phenomenologically, we have to work alone. Must we play the part, after all, of Husserl's 'solitary, individual philosophiser'? Is it not possible for phenomenological researchers to work with other people or to work as a team? Yes, it is possible. We need to note, all the same, that, in working with others and in working together, phenomenological researchers function in a fashion that is markedly different from the usual research pathways.

For a start, it will not be a matter of the phenomenological researcher gathering data in a straightforward manner from 'subjects' or 'respondents' and then analysing those data in some way or other, as happens in most other forms of social research. At the present time, it is politically correct to refer to the sources of data as co-researchers rather than subjects or respondents and to assert their equality with the principal researcher. In many instances this is little more than rhetoric and in some cases it is clearly no more than rhetoric. In phenomenological research, however, co-researchership has to be a genuine feature of the process for it to be phenomenological research at all.

Thus, each person involved must engage in phenomenological seeing in relation to her or his own experience. True enough, others can help. They can offer guidance as the person seeks to lay aside established notions and have a fresh look at the reality being encountered. As this person describes what has come into view, others can challenge what is being said to ensure its phenomenological and essential character. *What is it in the phenomenon as such that makes you say that? ... Are you importing the notion from the traditional understanding of this phenomenon? ... Would the phenomenon still be this phenomenon if this feature were absent? ...* Furthermore, other members of the group can compare and contrast this person's description of the phenomenon with what emerges for them when they themselves focus on their experience of the same phenomenon. Yes, there are many ways in which people can collaborate with individual co-researchers in the group. But they cannot do phenomenological research for them or on their behalf.

In this sense at least, though not necessarily in any professional or academic sense, everyone involved in phenomenological research has to be a phenomenologist. This being so, the co-researchers need to be hand-picked, for not everyone is equal to the task. In an earlier chapter we noted the great care with which van Kaam chose apt subjects for his study of the phenomenon of 'being understood'. We might also recall Spiegelberg's warning that the phenomenological task calls for 'a considerable degree of aptitude'.

This is already an indication that phenomenological research is likely to proceed along different lines from other forms of research. Elsewhere there is often emphasis on randomness in selecting subjects for research so as not to bias the sample and to ensure some degree of representativeness. Here no one is really representative of anything other than common, everyday human experience and the phenomena that enter that experience. In choosing people to work with phenomenologically, what we need to be concerned about is their ability to reflect, focus, intuit and describe as the phenomenological endeavour requires. They should be people who can put themselves in touch with their own immediate experience — disciplined people, therefore, who can prescind from their day-to-day, taken-for-granted assumptions, understandings and commitments and open themselves to the phenomena as these present themselves.

Doing phenomenology of this kind contrasts with the straightforward recording of subjective feelings, attitudes and perceptions that takes place in the new phenomenology. In an earlier chapter we noted that, in Spiegelberg's view, 'the "merely subjective" observations which characterize the reports of uncritical and untrained observers chosen at random' do not constitute phenomenological description. Also to be noted is Spiegelberg's further comment — a trenchant comment, surely — that phenomenology is 'definitely opposed' to the kind of subjectivism inherent in such observations and reports.[62]

It will be no easy matter to assemble a research team whose members can move freely from the noetic to the noematic, from the 'experiencing' to 'what is experienced'. If we wish to do a phenomenology of nursing, for instance, there will be little difficulty in finding nurses who are ready to talk about their feelings and attitudes towards nursing and the understandings they have of nursing. They will gladly tell how they love nursing or hate nursing, how they derive immense satisfaction and fulfilment from nursing or find nursing frustrating and alienating, how they approve of what is happening in nursing today or want to change the direction nursing is taking, how they have this understanding of nursing or that understanding of nursing. In all this they are describing themselves. It is another matter entirely to have them describe not themselves loving or hating nursing but *what is there* that they experience before any loving or hating ... not themselves fulfilled or frustrated by nursing but *what is there* that they experience before any sense of fulfilment or feeling of frustration ... not themselves approving or disapproving of nursing but *what is there* that they experience before giving approval or expressing disapproval ... not themselves understanding nursing in this way or that way but *what is there* that they experience before they attach any understandings to it at all. To find nurses who will focus on the phenomenon of nursing in that way and can describe nursing as it presents itself to them in their immediate experience of it is easier said than done.

Putting such a team together will not be helped by the fact that so many people today, including many nurses, are totally convinced that subjective feelings, personal attitudes and individual perceptions are the things that count anyway. This mindset has been fostered by much of what has come to the fore in humanistic psychology and the human potential movement it served to inform. It derives encouragement and support from writers like Carl Rogers,[63] who directs me, in my search for knowledge, to what I find 'within myself — from my own internal frame of reference'.

> I may 'know' that I love or hate, sense, perceive, comprehend. I may believe or disbelieve, enjoy or dislike, be interested in or bored by ... It is only by reference to the flow of feelings in me that I can begin to conceptualize an answer ... I taste a foreign dish. Do I like it? It is only by referring to the flow of my experiencing that I can sense the implicit meanings.[64]

The reality Rogers directs me to in this fashion is an inner reality. He is referring to what he calls 'subjective' knowledge — a way of knowing that relates to one's own inner states and derives from one's internal frame of reference. As we have seen in an earlier chapter, this is one of three forms of knowledge that Rogers distinguishes. There is also an 'objective' way of knowing that is validated by observation of external operations or from the reactions of a trustworthy reference group. Our third way of knowing is what Rogers calls 'interpersonal' or 'phenomenological' and it derives from our empathy-based entry into the private world of other individuals.

While he sees subjective knowledge as only one of three ways of knowing, for Rogers it is 'the most basic way of knowing'. It is a kind of organismic sensing. It stands over against objective knowledge, which founds 'all logical positivism, operationalism, and the vast structure of science as we know it'. Here human being and world are separated and opposed and tied to different ways of knowing. In human terms, as Rogers sees it, knowledge of the world may serve utilitarian purposes, but it is knowledge of my inner flow of experiencing that really counts.

What is missing in all this is the notion of intentionality so central to the phenomenological stance. Intentionality brings human being and world together and holds them together indissolubly. As Brentano led the way in emphasising, if I 'love' 'hate', 'sense', 'perceive' or 'comprehend', my love or hate are love and hate of *something*; I am sensing, perceiving, comprehending *something*. 'Husserl', Luijpen reminds us, 'conceived consciousness (knowledge) as intentionality — as orientation to what is not consciousness itself.'[65] In more existentialist terms, intentionality relates me essentially to the world.[66] I am not just a being with an inner world to explore.[67] I am a being-in-the-world, unable to be defined apart from the world just as my world cannot be defined apart from me. As a free, self-conscious being-in-the-world, I am destined to address that world, make sense of it and act upon it — to shape it even as I am shaped by it. The starting point, from the viewpoint of existential phenomenology, is to see the world as it presents itself to me and not merely as I have been taught to see it. If the research team is to engage in phenomenological research, its members must be able to throw off the excessive subjectivism that has become endemic in our kind of society so as to focus on the phenomena that are pre-given in our experience of the world.

Those team members will need to be hardy creatures. Phenomenological seeing does not come easily, even to those well and truly imbued with a phenomenological way of viewing things. To identify and delineate the essential phenomenon and make sure that its description is free of extraneous considerations, the researchers will need to return to their experience many times over. They may need to be *led back* to their experience many times over. Phenomenological researchers will do well to list patience and persistence as prominent weapons in their armoury.

Patient and persistent this work may need to be, but there are ample rewards to be gleaned from it. To lay aside old meanings is to open ourselves to new meanings or, at the very least, to bring new life to the meanings we hold. To break the bonds of 'mind-forg'd manacles' is to enjoy a new kind of freedom. To see the world with fresh eyes is to discover a whole new world.

NOTES

1 Marton (1986), p. 40.
2 Hardison (1989), pp. xii–xiii.
3 Natanson (1974), p. 60.
4 Wild (1955), pp. 191–192.
5 Gillan (1973), p. 8.
6 *Ibid.*, p. 15.
7 *Ibid.*, p. 7.
8 Husserl (1931), p. 43.
9 Merleau-Ponty (1962), p. 58.
10 Wild (1955), p. 192.
11 Spiegelberg (1982), p. 689.
12 May (1991), p. 26.
13 Malinowski (1948). pp. 100–101.
14 See Spiegelberg (1982), p. 146.
15 Heidegger (1977c), p. 303.
16 Kaufmann (1960), p. 273.
17 Heidegger (1959), p. 26.
18 van Manen (1990), p. 13.
19 Hawkes (1977), p. 62.
20 Bogdan (1990), p. 116.
21 Hawkes (1977), p. 62.
22 Merleau-Ponty (1962), p. xxi.
23 Geertz (1965), p. 668.
24 Langer (1953), p. 49.

25 *Ibid.*, p. 50.
26 Robinson (1987), p. 14.
27 See Rich (1990).
28 Sadler (1969), p. 377.
29 'Bracketing, like surrender, is no monopoly of phenomenologists or philosophers, nor of any other in any way special people. It may just *happen*, and to anybody — when one's received ideas do not function or no longer function but are, precisely, called into question. When may such an event occur? When may our traditional, habitual, customary methods fail? Any time — but perhaps it is possible to name typical situations in which it is more likely than in others; let us subsume them under the general label 'extreme situation', in the many meanings of this term. Among these meanings of 'extreme situation' is deep confusion, the unshakeable grip by something new, the feeling that everything is a riddle, that there is no sense to the world … It may be then that instead of continuing confusion or anxiety, there is a beginning of astonishment — of astonishment or wonderment which is the ever new-found root of philosophizing.' (Wolff 1984, pp. 194–195)
30 Kazantzakis (1959), p. 228.
31 Merleau-Ponty (1962), p. xiii.
32 Spiegelberg (1982), pp. 245–246.
33 See Schachtel (1963), pp. 279–322.
34 *Ibid.*, p. 288.
35 Scheler, in describing phenomenology as a 'psychic technique of non-resistance', also draws a contrast with Western thinking, i.e. with the combative stance towards the world to be found in the Western heroic attitude. See Stikkers (1985), esp. p. 136.
36 Cited in Spiegelberg (1982), p. 280.
37 Heidegger (1962), p. 206.
38 Heidegger (1977a), p. 112.
39 Levin (1989), p. 17.
40 Marcel (1965), p. 128.
41 Marcel (1964), p. 176.
42 See Marcel (1963), pp. 82–83.
43 Levinas (1967), p. 139.
44 See Percy (1990).
45 *Ibid.*, p. 463.
46 *Ibid.*, p. 464.
47 Gendlin (1965), p. 250.
48 Kullman and Taylor (1969), p. 120.
49 Merleau-Ponty (1962), p. 193.
50 Heidegger (1962), p. 63.
51 Frankl (1968), pp. 72–73. See also Frankl's definition of phenomenology: 'Phenomenology, as I understand it, speaks the language of man's prereflective self-understanding rather than interpreting a given phenomenon after preconceived patterns.' (*Ibid.*, p. 2).
52 See Ihde (1973).
53 O'Neill (1974), p. lxi.
54 'Much phenomenological description is compelled to use metaphor, to hint, "gesture" and "point" rather than clearly state, to surround its formulations with reservations and qualifications; all this because it is … largely concerned with what is given in pre-reflective (and pre-predicative) experience.' (Dunlop 1979, p. 70)
55 Marcel (1952), p. 299.

56 Kaelin (1965), p. 33.
57 Natanson (1977), pp. 112–113.
58 See Gendlin (1965).
59 See Bogdan (1990), *passim*.
60 See Godzich (1983), pp. xx–xxi.
61 In phenomenology, far from being presented as a source in which we discover phenomena, the understandings embedded in everyday accounts are portrayed as barriers: they are 'masks', 'blindfolds' and 'screens' that hide phenomena from us. Removing those barriers can only be done by the person concerned, so that phenomenological inquiry is inescapably a first-person exercise. Many otherwise perceptive writers on phenomenological inquiry fail to recognise this. Thus, van Manen talks of 'borrowing' other people's experiences and their reflections on their experiences' (1900, p. 62). Similarly, in his more recent work (1994), Moustakas looks to accounts given by respondents to provide 'textural' descriptions. 'From the textural descriptions, structural descriptions and an integration of textures and structures into the meanings and essences of the phenomenon are constructed' (pp. 118–119). As we have seen, however, phenomena are not constructed but intuited, and the intuiting can be done only by the subject of the experience. In this kind of inquiry we cannot 'borrow' other people's data.
62 Spiegelberg (1982), p. 689.
63 See Rogers (1969).
64 *Ibid.*, p. 23.
65 Luijpen (1969), pp. 33–34.
66 'We are involved in the world and with others in an inextricable tangle.' (Merleau-Ponty 1962, p. 454)
67 'This phenomenal field is not an "inner world", the "phenomenon" is not a "state of consciousness", or a "mental fact" ... Thus what we discover by going beyond the prejudice of the objective world is not an occult inner world.' (*Ibid.*, pp. 57–58).

Epilogue: Towards a phenomenology of nursing

Her name is Sharnee.

She sits at the end of the bed, behind her large, slanted table with all its columns and charts and figures.

Her eyes are constantly on the move. From one drip to the next. To the oxygen equipment. To the monitoring apparatus. Back to the broad sheet of paper on the table before her.

From time to time a warning sounds from one or other piece of equipment. She goes to it, examines it closely, turns off the warning device — and resumes her seat.

From time to time she approaches the person in the bed, changing his position and moving his arms and legs. A little while ago she removed the oxygen mask and rinsed his mouth out.

Now she is back at her table at the foot of the bed, busily writing on her charts and lists.

This is Intensive Care. And Sharnee is the nurse.

The man in the bed, deep in coma, is my friend, Sean. I keep vigil by his side as he is nursed through the night. And, in the course of this long watching and waiting, I find myself asking what's going on. Sharnee's a nurse. What's going on is nursing. So what is it? What is it that makes nursing nursing?

Oh, yes, I know what the textbooks have to say about it. 'Nursing is caring and caring is nursing', someone once said (Madeleine Leininger, wasn't it?). But, for my purposes here, that's the sort of thing I'm to ignore. I need to disregard it as far as I can. Put it aside. Simply focus on nursing as a phenomenon experienced here and now. 'Back to the things themselves!' And the thing itself I'm concerned with is nursing.

Not that it's so hard to forget about 'caring'. It's such a weasel word. Means anything and everything. What was I reading in that article the other day? The usual rhetoric about nursing being a matter of caring. Then the author went on to quote someone or other who had defined caring as helping persons to realise their full potential. So, our author concluded with rather triumphant logic, nursing is about helping people to reach their full potential. Ergo! QED!

I've always had problems with this 'full potential' business. My son wasn't any help either. It was some years ago and he was still at primary school. Sports Night was coming up and the event was to be graced with the presence of a local sporting celebrity, who at that time was appearing on our TV screens under the auspices of the Christian Television Association. Her message was along the lines, 'We all have God-given talents and our job is to realise these to the full.' My son said he was planning to have a word with her at the Sports Night. He was going to tell her he had outstanding potential as ... an assassin! All bravado, of course. He never did say a word to her. But you've got to admit he had a point. We all have such a vast range of potential — negative, destructive potential just as much as the more desirable kind. Which do we realise and which do we leave unrealised? What was it someone once said? That on our death bed we'll be able to look back and think about all the different lives we might have led; yet we will have lived only one of them.

That's not the only problem with this realisation-of-full-potential tack. What kind of thought process is it where we say that nursing means caring and then simply import a meaning for caring from an area totally unrelated to nursing? How valid a process is that? If one can import a meaning from X who says that caring means helping people to realise their full potential, what about Scott? Scott's my plumber. He has 'PLUMBING CARE' emblazoned on the side of his van when he comes to clear the sewerage pipes at my house. Shouldn't Scott get equal time?

Sean moves restlessly in the bed and I feel a bit guilty about the direction my thoughts are taking. Hardly time for levity, is it. Levity? Hang on now ... But I suppress the urge to defend myself against the charge. It doesn't seem worth the effort. So I just try to disregard talk of 'caring' and see if there isn't a better word to describe nursing as it presents itself to me in my immediate experience of it.

What does nursing strike me as being? Well, right now 'support' is the word that springs to mind. What Sharnee is doing is supporting Sean, keeping him going, as his system does battle against the organisms in his lungs that threaten to end his life.

'Support'? Yes, it does seem to fit. I recall the brief conversation I had with Sharnee an hour or so ago. I was looking for reassurance. 'What's going to happen?'. I had asked her anxiously. "It's up to Sean now,' she replied gently. 'It's entirely up to Sean.'

Yes, it's up to Sean. Nursing can't heal him. It can only support him as, hopefully, he heals himself.

Snatches of another conversation with a nurse come back to me. It was a few weeks ago. I was talking with Maureen, a midwife, about her experiences in the labour ward. 'I've had plenty of experience in medical and surgical wards,' Maureen said, 'but midwifery is different.' She was making the point that in the labour ward. generally speaking, the nurse isn't dealing with sick people. She had actually drawn breath to talk about something else when she added, rather casually, 'Well, you know, when I come to think about it, I'm not so sure about that. Maybe it's not so different after all.'

It was almost an aside. Just a comment tossed off after that particular discussion had come to a close. By the time her words had assumed any importance in my mind, Maureen was well into a diatribe about the management at the Nursing School. 'Hey, Maureen, just a minute ... !'

Maureen was happy to explain. She had had an afterthought. It had suddenly come to her that midwifery work and nursing in the acute-care setting have more in common than one generally gives them credit for. 'I was telling you that the nurse deals with sick people in medical and surgical wards, whereas in the labour ward it's different. There you're dealing with people who, for the most part, are well. In midwifery, I was thinking, the nurse simply supports people while they do what they have to do and what no one else can do for them. But then it struck me that the nurse is doing very much the same thing in Acute Care too. There too, in the end, you're really supporting people as they do the work of healing themselves.'

'Support'. Yes, it does seem to square with what goes on in nursing. And 'support' can take many forms. It can extend appropriately to many different nursing contexts.

Or is that just another way of saying that 'support' too is a weasel word? Maybe all the unkind things I've been saying about 'care' can be equally levelled at 'support'! Hoist with my own petard!

On second thoughts, perhaps not. Support may take many forms but the basic meaning of the word persists. Unlike 'care', which has so many meanings. 'Care' lends itself to the very Christian concept of responding with compassion to human need. It can embrace the more emotion-laden notion of 'being fond of'. And it stretches all the way to Heidegger's Sorge, which has to do merely with our dealing with things, our basic involvement in the world. No, I don't think 'support' is a word like that.

'Support' certainly doesn't carry the sentimental overtones of the word 'care'. Not that I have anything against sentiment. Nor am I overlooking the merit in, say, Anselm Strauss's characterisation of certain aspects of nursing as 'sentimental work'. Still, as I look about the intensive care ward tonight, there doesn't seem to be much place for sentiment. Care, understood as interpersonal relationship, looms large in nursing theory but, in the case of Sean and Sharnee, where is there interpersonal relationship in any true sense of the term? How could there be? Sean has been unconscious since he was brought here. And Sharnee's attention seems to be directed far more to the technology surrounding Sean in such complex abundance than to Sean himself. Curiously, I find myself feeling very thankful

that it is. I have a deep sense that, were Sharnee to be experiencing any kind of interpersonal relationship to Sean at this moment, it could very well prove a distraction and a hindrance. Better that she feel a clinical detachment that allows her to concentrate fully on her complicated tasks. Better, in that sense at least, that she support rather than care.

Strange that. For all the talk about nursing being caring, with caring cast in terms that are not even possible for Sharnee in these circumstances, she strikes me nonetheless as a superb nurse. She is providing Sean with the very best kind of support in the best kind of way. (If I'm ever in Intensive Care myself, that's the support I'd like to get — and Sharnee's the type of nurse I'd want at the end of my bed!)

Yes, indeed, nurses support their clients. At all times and in all kinds of ways. Nursing strikes me as being such total support. It supports the whole person. To use what is already an overused word, the support it gives is holistic.

As I sit in hospital wards and community health centres, I see many professionals at work. Podiatrists. Speech therapists. Physiotherapists. Psychologists. Occupational therapists. Doctors. Their role seems so much more focused. On clients' feet. On their tongue and facial muscles. On a particular injury or disability or overall motor skills. On emotional problems. On involvement with particular activities or the development of particular skills. On treatment of illness. In comparison, the nurse's role seems so totally without focus. Even in the more regimented hospital setting this is apparent. At one moment, monitoring body temperature, blood pressure and the pulse rate; at another, emptying the ileostomy bag. At one moment, administering medications; at another, providing important information to the patient. At one moment, collecting a bed pan; at another moment, or perhaps at the same moment, stopping to chat and allay a patient's anxiety with some skilful 'active listening'. Add to that the patient advocacy and action-for-change that are emerging today as essential nursing roles. What can the nurse not be called upon to do in support of nursing clients? The support nurses give is total support and it serves to distinguish them from many other health professionals.

Sitting by Sean's bedside in Intensive Care, I find a phrase used by Heidegger coming to my mind, as it has at many other times when I've been observing nurses at work. 'The nursing of the sick body'. When I first read those words in Being and Time, they seemed to have an old-fashioned ring to them. Yet, tonight, as always, the reference to the body appears so pivotal. When I see chaplains and counsellors at the bedside of the sick, I know at once that they're not nurses — and it has nothing to do with the wearing of a clerical collar or the non-wearing of a uniform . The central reason why they're clearly not nursing their clients is their primary focus on 'souls' or 'psyches' rather than 'bodies'. If saying that does less than justice to a genuinely holistic viewpoint, I'll gladly rephrase it: they're clearly not nursing because their chief focus is on the spiritual or the psychological rather than the somatic.

I find myself being careful to add words like 'primary' or 'chief' here when I talk to myself about the focus of these professionals. There is nothing in their *perceived relationship with their clients to suggest that they are failing to work within a holistic perspective. I'm not suggesting that the priest who came in to see Sean this afternoon saw him as a pure spirit. And the counsellor who spoke with Sean's wife certainly didn't treat her like some disembodied mind. For all that, their role didn't strike me as being particularly somatic.*

In contrast, the nursing role as experienced does seem essentially somatic. It seems so very bodily in its primary orientation. Nurses do such bodily things. One just can't avoid seeing nursing clients, and therefore the nurses themselves, as first and foremost embodied beings.

Importantly, that bodily dimension provides a context for all other aspects of nursing. Nurses too do their share of counselling and consoling and inspiring. But, in their case, such services always seem to be coloured by an overall context of bodily attention paid to the patient. Where that context is absent, it may be a nurse doing the counselling and consoling and inspiring, but it is not experienced as nursing. It is experienced, instead, as counselling or pastoral care by someone who happens to be a nurse. (And, from the phenomenological perspective, how something is experienced is of paramount importance. For us, in our knowledge of things, the ultimate court of appeal lies in our very experience of them. Merleau-Ponty tells us that somewhere or other, doesn't he?)

The bodiliness is always there in the case of nursing. It is not there in the same way in the psychotherapy offered by the counsellor or the spiritual guidance provided by the chaplain. So, as I observe nursing as immediately as I can and ask myself how it presents itself to me, it emerges for me very much as a body-centred way of relating.

Nurses — and nursing clients — as embodied beings. As I reflect on my experience in this respect, I find myself very aware that being embodied means far more than just having a body. In my experience of people being nursed, they don't appear merely as people who have *bodies. Rather, they* are *their bodies. Modern health care has been criticised very harshly, and no doubt justly, for its overemphasis on physical causes, physical symptoms and physical outcomes. Nursing has borne its share of such criticism. Fingers have been pointed at nurses' Coronary-in-Bed-6 attitude. But that kind of attitude stems from a reductionist approach. It is a perspective wherein the physical is separated from the psychosocial and the spiritual and from the totality of the person. When nursing impresses itself upon me as being somatic in its primary focus, there is no separation of that kind. The psychosocial and the spiritual are not overlooked or downgraded. They are well and truly there. They are genuinely taken account of. They are simply given a context, an horizon. And the context is bodiliness; the horizon is embodiment.*

Nursing as support. Nursing as total-person in scope. Nursing as body-centred in focus. Nursing seems to be assuming a certain structure in my experience of it, doesn't it? And, at least with these dimensions coming together in the way they do, there seems to be a shape to my description of it that is not hugely prominent in treatises of nursing theory.

Of course, I'm doing something quite different from what the authors do in their treatises on nursing theory. I'm certainly meant to be doing something quite different. I'm not meant to be reasoning about what nursing is. I'm meant to be reflecting on the experience of nursing and delineating what it is, in that very experience and for no other reason, that leads me as observer to say, 'Yes, that is nursing', or makes the nurse say, 'Yes, I really am nursing', or causes the client to say, 'Yes, I am indeed being nursed.'

What, then, am I up to here? Have I begun a phenomenology of nursing? As I continue these musings at Sean's bedside, I can think of one author who might very well want to say that I am presenting phenomenal findings rather than doing a full-on phenomenology. Yet another author comes to mind who would almost certainly be muttering something like, 'Loose but intuitively interesting flitting across an experiential theme.' And now an image of Max Scheler is looming before me: Max is smiling his wry smile and saying, 'This is what I meant by "picture-book phenomenology"!'

OK, I'll make no great claims for these musings of mine. Maybe I should borrow a leaf from Winston Churchill's book. 'This is not the end. It is not even the beginning of the end. But it is, perhaps, the end of the beginning.' I need to move on. Not, to be sure, by reasoning about what I've encountered and what has emerged for me from the encounter. (What was it Heidegger said? About reason, 'glorified for centuries', being 'the most stiff-necked adversary of thought'?) No, I'll move on, paradoxically, by going back. For I need to return again and again to what I've encountered and encounter it anew. I need to surrender to it more thoroughly, contemplate it more deeply, listen to it more attentively. It has begun to assume a certain structure in my experience of it; I need to allow that structure to emerge in ever sharper relief. In particular, I need to ask myself — and others — not whether this emerging picture of nursing squares at all with nursing history or nursing traditions or nursing theories, but whether I'm allowing the phenomenon of nursing to present itself to me as directly as possible ... whether I'm describing it as best I can without regard to inherited and prevailing understandings of nursing ... yes, and whether, as just a start at phenomenological seeing, it has been worth the effort.

Bibliography

Ainlay, S C (1983). 'Intentionality and the investigation of the social world'. *Current Perspectives in Social Theory* 4, pp. 3–22.

Anderson, J M (1991a). 'Immigrant women speak of chronic illness: the social construction of the devalued self'. *Journal of Advanced Nursing* 16:6 (June), pp. 710–717.

Anderson, J M. (1991b). 'Current directions in nursing research: toward a poststructuralist and feminist epistemology'. *The Canadian Journal of Nursing Research* 23:3 (Fall), pp. 1–3.

Armstrong, E G (1976). 'On phenomenology and sociological theory'. *British Journal of Sociology* 27:2 (June 1976), pp. 251–253.

Arnett, R C and Nakagawa, G (1983). 'The assumptive roots of empathic listening: a critique'. *Communication Education* 32 (October), pp. 368–378.

Baker, C, Wuest, J and Stern, P N (1992). 'Method slurring: the grounded theory/phenomenology example'. *Journal of Advanced Nursing* 17:11 (November), pp. 1355–1360.

Bauman, Z (1973). 'On the philosophical status of ethnomethodology'. *The Sociological Review* 21 (February 1973), pp. 5–23.

Bauman, Z (1976). *Towards a Critical Sociology: An Essay on Commonsense and Emancipation.* London: Routledge & Kegan Paul.

Beck, C T (1991a). 'How students perceive faculty caring: a phenomenological study'. *Nurse Educator* 16:5 (September-October), pp. 18–22.

Beck, C T (1991b). 'Undergraduate nursing students' lived experience of health: a phenomenological study'. *Journal of Nursing Education* 30:8 (October), pp. 371–374.

Beck, C T (1992). 'The lived experience of postpartum depression: a phenomenological study'. *Nursing Research* 41:3 (May-June), pp. 166–170.

Bedford, E (1989). 'Empiricism'. In *The Concise Encyclopedia of Western Philosophy and Philosophers*, revised edition, eds J O Urmson and J Rée, London: Routledge, pp. 88–90.

Benner, P (1984). *From Novice to Expert: Excellence and Power in Clinical Nursing Practice.* Menlo Park, Calif: Addison-Wesley.

Benner, P (1985). 'Quality of life: a phenomenological perspective on explanation, prediction, and understanding in nursing science'. *Advances in Nursing Science* 8:1, pp. 1–14.

Benner, P and Wrubel, J (1989). *The Primacy of Caring: Stress and Coping in Health and Illness*. Menlo Park, Calif: Addison-Wesley.

Bennett, L (1991). 'Adolescent girls' experience of witnessing marital violence: a phenomenological study'. *Journal of Advanced Nursing* 16:4 (April), pp. 431–438.

Bernstein, R J (1991). *The New Constellation: The Ethical-Political Horizons of Modernity/Postmodernity*. Oxford: Polity Press.

Binswanger, L (1963). *Being-in-the-World*. New York: Basic Books.

Bochenski, I M (1974). *Contemporary European Philosophy*. Berkeley: University of California Press.

Boelen, B (1975). 'Martin Heidegger as a phenomenologist'. In *Phenomenological Perspectives: Historical and Systematic Essays in Honor of Herbert Spiegelberg*, ed. P J Bossert, The Hague: Martinus Nijhoff, pp. 93–114.

Bogdan, D (1990). 'In and out of love with literature'. In Part II 'The phenomenology of reading', *Beyond Communication: Reading Comprehension and Criticism*, eds D Bogdan and S B Straw, Portsmouth, NH: Boynton/Cook, pp. 109–137.

Bossert, P J (1985). '"Plato's cave", *Flatland* and Phenomenology'. In *Phenomenology in Practice and Theory*, ed. W S Hamrick, The Hague: Martinus Nijhoff, pp. 53–66.

Bourne, R (1977). *The Radical Will: Selected Writings 1911–1918*, ed. O Hansen, New York: Urizen Books.

Bowman, J M (1991). 'The meaning of chronic low back pain'. *AAOHN Journal* 39:8 (August), pp. 381–384.

Breault, A J and Polifroni, E C (1992). 'Caring for people with AIDS: nurses' attitudes and feelings'. *Journal of Advanced Nursing* 17:1 (January), pp. 21–27.

Brentano, F (1973). *Psychology from an Empirical Standpoint*. London: Routledge & Kegan Paul.

Buber, M (1958). *I and Thou*. 2nd edition. New York: Charles Scribner's Sons.

Buber, M (1966). *The Knowledge of Man: A Philosophy of the Interhuman*. New York: Harper & Row.

Caputo, J D (1993). 'Heidegger and theology'. In *The Cambridge Companion to Heidegger*, ed. C B Guignon, Cambridge: Cambridge University Press, pp. 270–288.

Cicourel, A (1968). *The Social Organization of Juvenile Justice*. New York: Wiley.

Cohen, M Z (1987). 'A historical overview of the phenomenologic movement'. *Image: Journal of Nursing Scholarship* 19:1 (Spring), pp. 31–34.

Colaizzi, P (1978). 'Psychological research as the phenomenologist views it'. In *Existential-Phenomenological Alternatives for Psychology*, eds R Valle and M King, New York: Oxford University Press, pp. 48–71.

Demske, J M (1970). *Being, Man and Death: A Key to Heidegger*. Lexington: University Press of Kentucky.

Denzin, N K (1978). 'The methodological implications of symbolic interactionism for the study of deviance'. In *Contemporary Social Theories*, ed. A Wells, Santa Monica: Goodyear, pp. 99–108.

Derrida, J (1991). 'Philosopher's hell: an interview'. In *The Heidegger Controversy: A Critical Reader*, ed. R Wolin, New York: Columbia University Press, pp. 245–263.

Dewey, J (1925). *Experience and Nature*. Chicago: Open Court.

Diekelmann, N L (1992). 'Learning-as-testing: a Heideggerian hermeneutical analysis of the lived experiences of students and teachers in nursing'. *Advances in Nursing Science* 14:3 (March), pp. 72–83.

Dobbie, B J (1991). 'Women's mid-life experience: an evolving consciousness of self and children'. *Journal of Advanced Nursing* 16:7 (July), pp. 825–831.

Douglas, J D (1974). *Defining America's Social Problems*. Englewood Cliffs, NJ: Prentice-Hall.

Douglass, B J and Moustakas, C (1985). 'Heuristic inquiry: the internal search to know'. *Journal of Humanistic Psychology* 25:3 (Summer), pp. 39–55.

Dreyfus, H L (ed.) (1982). *Husserl, Intentionality and Cognitive Science*. Cambridge, Mass: MIT Press.

Dunlop, F (1979). 'Phenomenology and education'. *Journal of Further and Higher Education* 3:2 (Summer), pp. 67–77.

Edie, J M (1964). 'Introduction'. In M Merleau-Ponty, *Primacy of Perception, and other essays*, Evanston: Northwestern University Press, pp. xiii–xix.

Elfert, H, Anderson, J M and Lai, M (1991). 'Parents' perceptions of children with chronic illness: a study of immigrant Chinese families'. *Journal of Pediatric Nursing* 6:2 (April), pp. 114–120.

Emad, P (1972). 'Max Scheler's phenomenology of shame'. *Philosophy and Phenomenological Research* 3 (March), pp. 361–370.

Eyres, S J, Loustau, A and Ersek, M (1992). 'Ways of knowing among beginning students in nursing'. *Journal of Nursing Education* 31:4 (April), pp. 175–180.

Farías, V (1989). *Heidegger and Nazism*. Philadelphia: Temple University Press.

Fell, J P (1979). *Heidegger and Sartre: An Essay on Being and Place*. New York: Columbia University Press.

Frankl, V E (1968). *Psychotherapy and Existentialism: Selected Papers on Logotherapy*. New York: Simon & Schuster.

Friedman, M (1964). 'Introduction'. In *The Worlds of Existentialism: A Critical Reader*, ed. M Friedman, New York: Random House, pp. 3–14.

Gallant, M J and Kleinman, S (1983). 'Symbolic interactionism vs. ethno-methodology'. *Symbolic Interaction* 6:1, pp. 1–18.

Garfinkel, H (1967). *Studies in Ethnomethodology*. Englewood Cliffs, NJ: Prentice-Hall.

Geertz, C (1965). 'Religion as a cultural system'. Chapter 18 in *The Religious Situation*, ed. D R Cutler, Boston: Beacon Press, pp. 639–688.

Gendlin, E T (1965). 'Expressive meanings'. In *An Invitation to Phenomenology: Studies in the Philosophy of Experience*, ed. James M Edie, Chicago: Quadrangle Books, pp. 240–251.

Giddens, A (1989). *Sociology*. Cambridge: Polity Press.

Gillan, G (1973). 'In the folds of the flesh: philosophy and language'. Chapter 1 in *Horizons of the Flesh: Critical Perspectives on the Thought of Merleau-Ponty*, ed. G Gillan, Carbondale: Illinois University Press, pp. 1–60.

Giorgi, A (1970). *Psychology as a Human Science: A Phenomenologically Based Approach*. New York: Harper & Row.

Giorgi, A (1971). 'Phenomenology and experimental psychology'. In *Duquesne Studies in Phenomenological Psychology*, Vol. I, eds A Giorgi, W Fischer and R van Eckartsberg, Pittsburgh: Duquesne University Press, pp. 7–15.

Giorgi, A (1975a). 'Convergence and divergence of qualitative and quantitative method in psychology'. *In Duquesne Studies in Phenomenological Psychology*, Vol. II, eds A Giorgi, C T Fisher and E L Murray, Pittsburgh: Duquesne University Press, pp. 71–79.

Giorgi, A (1975b). 'An application of the phenomenological method in psychology'. In *Duquesne Studies in Phenomenological Psychology*, Vol. II, eds A Giorgi, C T Fisher and E L Murray, Pittsburgh: Duquesne University Press, pp. 82–103.

Giorgi, A (1985). 'Sketch of a psychological phenomenological method'. In *Phenomenology and Psychological Research*, ed. A Giorgi, Pittsburgh: Duquesne University Press, pp. 8–22.

Godzich, W (1983). 'Caution! Reader at work!' Introduction to *Blindness and Insight: Essay on the Rhetoric of Contemporary Criticism*, ed. P de Man, 2nd edition, Minneapolis: University of Minnesota Press, pp. xv–xxx.

Gorman, R A (1977). *The Dual Vision: Alfred Schutz and the Myth of Phenomenological Social Science*. London: Routledge & Kegan Paul.

Gortner, S R and Schultz, P R (1988). 'Approaches to nursing science methods'. *Image: Journal of Nursing Scholarship* 20:1 (Spring), pp. 22–24.

Grene, M (1960). *Introduction to Existentialism*. Chicago: University of Chicago Press.

Grossberg, L (1983). 'The phenomenological challenge in sociology'. In *Foundations of Morality, Human Rights, and the Human Sciences: Phenomenology in a Foundational Dialogue with the Human Sciences*, eds A T Tymieniecka and C O Schrag, Boston: Reidel, pp. 99–118.

Guignon, C B (1993). 'Introduction'. In *The Cambridge Companion to Heidegger*, ed. C B Guignon, Cambridge: Cambridge University Press, pp. 1–41.

Gurwitsch, A. (1966). *Studies in Phenomenology and Psychology*. Evanston: Northwestern University Press.

Gurwitsch, A. (1967). 'Intentionality, constitution, and intentional analysis'. In *Phenomenology: The Philosophy of Edmund Husserl and Its Interpretation*, ed. J J Kockelmans, New York: Doubleday, pp. 118–149.

Habermas, J (1991). 'Martin Heidegger: On the publication of the lectures of 1935'. In *The Heidegger Controversy: A Critical Reader*, ed. R Wolin, New York: Columbia University Press, pp. 186–197.

Hammond, M, Howarth, J and Keat, R (1991). *Understanding Phenomenology*. Cambridge, Mass: Basil Blackwell.

Hardin, J B, Power, M B and Sugrue, N M (1986). 'The progressive concretization of phenomenological sociology'. *Studies in Symbolic Interaction* 7A, pp. 49–74.

Hardison, O B (Jr) (1989). *Disappearing through the Skylight: Culture and Technology in the Twentieth Century*. New York: Penguin.

Harries, K (1978). 'Heidegger as a political thinker'. In *Heidegger and Modern Philosophy: Critical Essays*, ed. M Murray, New Haven: Yale University Press, pp. 304–328.

Harvey, M (1972). 'Sociological theory: the production of a bourgeois ideology'. In *Counter Course: A Handbook for Course Criticism*, ed. T Pateman, Harmondsworth: Penguin, pp. 82–111.

Hauck, M R (1991). 'Mothers' descriptions of the toilet-training process: a phenomenologic study'. *Journal of Pediatric Nursing* 6:2 (April), pp. 80–86.

Hawkes, T (1977). *Structuralism and Semiotics*. London: Methuen.

Heap, J L and Roth, P A (1978). 'On phenomenological sociology'. In *Contemporary Sociological Theories*, ed. A Wells, Santa Monica: Goodyear, pp. 279–293.

Heidegger, M (1949a). 'Remembrance of the poet'. In *Existence and Being*, ed. W Brock, Chicago: Regnery, pp. 233–269.

Heidegger, M (1949b). 'What is metaphysics?'. In *Existence and Being*, ed. W Brock, Chicago: Regnery, pp. 353–392.

Heidegger, M (1949c). 'Hölderlin and the essence of poetry'. In *Existence and Being*, ed. W Brock, Chicago: Regnery, pp. 270–291.

Heidegger, M (1959). *An Introduction to Metaphysics*. New Haven: Yale University Press.

Heidegger, M (1962). *Being and Time*. Oxford: Basil Blackwell.

Heidegger, M (1971). *On the Way to Language*. New York: Harper & Row.

Heidegger, M (1975). *Poetry, Language, Thought*. New York: Harper Colophon.

Heidegger, M (1977a). 'What is metaphysics?' In *Martin Heidegger: Basic Writings*, ed. D F Krell, New York: Harper & Row, pp. 95–112.

Heidegger, M (1977b). 'Letter on humanism'. In *Martin Heidegger: Basic Writings*, ed. D F Krell, New York: Harper & Row, pp. 193–242.

Heidegger, M (1977c). 'The question concerning technology'. In *Martin Heidegger: Basic Writings*, ed. D F Krell, New York: Harper & Row, pp. 287–317.

Heidegger, M (1982). *The Basic Problems of Phenomenology*. Bloomington: Indiana University Press.

Heidegger, M (1989). *Beiträge zur Philosophie*. Vol. 65 in *Gesamtausgabe*, ed. F-W von Hermann, Frankfurt am Main: Klostermann.

Heidegger, M (1991a). 'The self-assertion of the German university'. In *The Heidegger Controversy: A Critical Reader*, ed. R Wolin, New York: Columbia University Press, pp. 29–39.

Heidegger, M (1991b). 'German students'. In *The Heidegger Controversy: A Critical Reader*, ed. R Wolin, New York: Columbia University Press, pp. 46–47.

Heidegger, M (1991c). '"Only a God can save us": *Der Spiegel*'s interview with Martin Heidegger (1966)'. In *The Heidegger Controversy: A Critical Reader*, ed. R Wolin, New York: Columbia University Press, pp. 91–116..

Henderson, A D — Brouse, A J (1991). 'The experiences of new fathers during the first three weeks of life'. *Journal of Advanced Nursing* 16:3 (March), pp. 293–298.

Heron, J (1970). 'The phenomenology of social encounter: the gaze'. *Philosophy and Phenomenological Research* 31, pp. 243–264.

Hindess, B (1992). 'Heidegger and the Nazis: cautionary tales of the relations between theory and practice'. *Thesis Eleven* 31, pp. 115–130.

Hoy, D C (1993). 'Heidegger and the hermeneutic turn'. In *The Cambridge Companion to Heidegger*, ed. C B Guignon, Cambridge: Cambridge University Press, pp. 170–194.

Husserl, E (1931). *Ideas: General Introduction to Pure Phenomenology*. London: George Allen & Unwin.

Husserl, E (1964). *The Idea of Phenomenology*. The Hague: Martinus Nijhoff.

Husserl, E (1965). *Phenomenology and the Crisis of Philosophy*. New York: Harper & Row.

Husserl, E (1970a). *Logical Investigations*. Vols I–II. London: Routledge & Kegan Paul.

Husserl, E (1970b). *The Crisis of European Sciences and Transcendental Phenomenology*. Evanston: Northwestern University Press.

Husserl, E (1970c). *Cartesian Meditations: An Introduction to Phenomenology*. The Hague: Martinus Nijhoff.

Husserl, E (1973). *Experience and Judgment: Investigations in a Genealogy of Logic*. Ed. L Landgrebe. London: Routledge & Kegan Paul.

Husserl, E (1981). 'Inaugural lecture at Freiburg im Breisgau'. In *Husserl: Shorter Works*, eds P McCormick and F Elliston, South Bend: University of Notre Dame Press, pp. 9–20.

Ihde, D (1973). 'Singing the world: language and perception'. Chapter 2 in *Horizons of the Flesh: Critical Perspectives on the Thought of Merleau-Ponty*, ed. G Gillan, Carbondale: Illinois University Press, pp. 61–77.

Islam, N (1983). 'Sociology, phenomenology and phenomenological sociology'. *Sociological Bulletin* 32:2 (September), pp. 137–152.

Kaelin, E F (1962). *An Existentialist Aesthetic: The Theories of Sartre and Merleau-Ponty*. Madison: University of Wisconsin Press.

Kaelin, E (1965). 'The visibility of things seen: a phenomenological view of painting'. In *An Invitation to Phenomenology: Studies in the Philosophy of Experience*, ed. James M Edie, Chicago: Quadrangle Books, pp. 30–58.

Kaelin, E F (1988). *Heidegger's* Being and Time*: A Reading for Readers*. Tallahassee: Florida State University Press.

Kaufmann, W (1960). *From Shakespeare to Existentialism*. 2nd edition. New York: Doubleday.

Kazantzakis, N (1959). *Zorba the Greek*. New York: Simon & Schuster.

Keefe, M R and Froese-Fretz, A (1991). 'Living with an irritable infant: maternal perspectives'. *MCN* 16:5 (September–October), pp. 255–259.

Kockelmans, J J (1965). *Martin Heidegger: A First Introduction to His Philosophy*. Pittsburgh: Duquesne University Press.

Kockelmans, J J (1967). *Phenomenology: The Philosophy of Edmund Husserl and Its Interpretation*. New York: Doubleday.

Kohak, E (1978). *Idea and Experience*. Chicago: University of Chicago Press.

Krell, D F (1989). 'Heidegger'. In *The Concise Encyclopedia of Western Philosophy and Philosophers*, revised edition, eds J O Urmson and J Rée, London: Routledge, pp. 128–130.

Kullman, M — Taylor, C (1969). 'The pre-objective world'. In *Essays in Phenomenology*, ed. M Natanson, The Hague: Martinus Nijhoff, pp. 116–136.

Langan, T (1966). *The Meaning of Heidegger: A Critical Study of an Existentialist Phenomenology*. New York: Columbia University Press.

Langer, S (1953). *Feeling and Form*. New York: Charles Scribner's Sons.

Lasch, C (1979). *The Culture of Narcissism*. New York: Norton.

Lavine, T Z (1990). 'Thinking like a Nazi: a review essay of Victor Farías, *Heidegger and Nazism*'. *International Journal of Group Tensions* 20:3 (Fall), pp. 279–285.

Leonard, V W (1989). 'A Heideggerian phenomenologic perspective on the concept of the person'. *Advances in Nursing Science* 11:4, pp. 40–55.

Lethbridge, D J (1991). 'Choosing and using contraception: toward a theory of women's contraceptive self-care'. *Nursing Research* 40:5 (September–October), pp. 276–280.

Levin, D M (1989). *The Listening Self: Personal Growth, Social Change and the Closure of Metaphysics*. London: Routledge.

Levinas, E (1967). 'Martin Buber and the theory of knowledge'. Chapter 5 in *The Philosophy of Martin Buber*, eds P A Schilpp and M Friedman, La Salle, Ill: Open Court, pp. 133–150.

Lewis, J (1975). *Max Weber and Value-Free Sociology: A Marxist Critique*. London: Lawrence & Wishart.

Löwith, K (1991). 'The political implications of Heidegger's existentialism'. In *The Heidegger Controversy: A Critical Reader*, ed. R Wolin, New York: Columbia University Press, pp. 167–185.

Luegenbiehl, H C (1976). *The Essence of Man: An Approach to the Philosophy of Martin Heidegger*. PhD dissertation. Ann Arbor: University Microfilms International.

Luijpen, W A (1969). *Existential Phenomenology*. 2nd edition. Pittsburgh: Duquesne University Press.

Macionis, J J (1991). *Sociology*. 3rd edition. Englewood Cliffs, NJ: Prentice Hall.

Mahrer, A R (1989). 'The case for fundamentally different existential-humanistic psychologies'. *Journal of Humanistic Psychology* 29:2 (Spring), pp. 249–262.

Malinowski, B (1948). *Magic, Science and Religion, and Other Essays*. London: Souvenir.

Marcel, G (1952). *Metaphysical Journal*. London: Rockliff.

Marcel, G (1963). *The Existential Background of Human Dignity*. Cambridge: Harvard University Press.

Marcel, G (1964). *Creative Fidelity*. New York: Farrar, Straus & Giroux.

Marcel, G (1965). *The Philosophy of Existentialism*. 5th edition. New York: Citadel.

Maritain, J (1959). *The Degrees of Knowledge*. London: Geoffrey Bles.

Marr, J (1991). 'The experience of living with Parkinson's disease'. *Journal of Neuroscience Nursing* 23:5 (October), pp. 325–329.

Martin, L S (1991). 'Using Watson's theory to explore the dimensions of adult polycystic kidney disease'. *ANNA Journal* 18:5 (October), pp. 493–496.

Marton, F (1986). 'Phenomenography: a research approach to investigating different understandings of reality'. *Journal of Thought* 21:3 (Fall), pp. 28–49.

Maslow, A H (1957). 'A philosophy of psychology: the need for a mature science of human nature'. *Main Currents in Modern Thought* 13, pp. 27–32.

Mason, C (1992). 'Non-attendance at out-patient clinics: a case study'. *Journal of Advanced Nursing* 17:5 (May), pp. 554–560.

Massarik, F (1981). 'The interviewing process re-examined'. In *Human Inquiry: A Sourcebook of New Paradigm Research*, eds P Reason and J Rowan, Chichester: Wiley & Sons, pp. 201–206.

May, R (1982). 'The problem of evil: an open letter to Carl Rogers'. *Journal of Humanistic Psychology* 22:3 (Summer), pp. 10–21.

May, R (1991). *The Cry for Myth*. London: Souvenir Press.

May, R, Angel, E and Ellenberger, H F (1958). *Existence: A New Dimension in Psychiatry and Psychology*. New York: Basic Books.

McCall, R J (1983). *Phenomenological Psychology: An Introduction*. Madison: University of Wisconsin Press.

McCleary, R C (1964). 'Translator's preface'. In M Merleau-Ponty, *Signs*, Evanston: Northwestern University Press, pp. ix–xxxii.

McHaffie, H E (1991). 'Neonatal intensive care units: visiting policies for grandparents'. *Midwifery* 7 (September), pp. 122–132.

Merleau-Ponty, M (1962). *Phenomenology of Perception*. London: Routledge & Kegan Paul.

Merleau-Ponty, M (1964a). *Sense and Non-Sense*. Evanston: Northwestern University Press.

Merleau-Ponty, M (1964b). *Signs*. Evanston: Northwestern University Press.

Merleau-Ponty, M (1964c). *Primacy of Perception, and other essays*. Evanston: Northwestern University Press.

Merleau-Ponty, M (1965). *The Structure of Behaviour*. London: Methuen.

Merleau-Ponty, M (1968). *The Visible and the Invisible*. Evanston: Northwestern University Press.

Misgeld, D (1983). 'Common sense and common convictions: sociology as a science, phenomenological sociology and the hermeneutical point of view'. *Human Studies* 6, pp. 109–139.

Misiak, H and Sexton, V S (1973). *Phenomenological, Existential, and Humanistic Psychologies: A Historical Survey*. New York: Grune & Stratton.

Mitchell, J C (1977). 'The logic and methods of sociological inquiry'. Chapter 2 in *Introducing Sociology*, ed. P Worsley, 2nd edition, Harmondsworth: Penguin, pp. 73–121.

Monahan, R S (1992). 'Nursing home employment: the nurse's aide's perspective'. *Journal of Gerontological Nursing* 18:2 (February), pp. 13–16.

Montbriand, M J — Laing, G P (1991). 'Alternative health care as a control strategy'. *Journal of Advanced Nursing* 16:3 (March), pp. 325–332.

Moore, A (1965). 'Existentialism and the tradition'. In *An Invitation to Phenomenology: Studies in the Philosophy of Experience*, ed. James M Edie, Chicago: Quadrangle Books, pp. 91–109.

Moustakas, C (1961). *Loneliness*. Englewood Cliffs, NJ: Prentice Hall.

Moustakas, C (1981). 'Heuristic research'. In *Human Inquiry: A Sourcebook of New Paradigm Research*, eds P Reason and J Rowan, Chichester: John Wiley & Sons.

Moustakas, C (1994). *Phenomenological Research Methods*. Thousand Oaks: Sage.

Mumford, L (1950). 'The pragmatic acquiescence'. In *Pragmatism and American Culture*, ed. G Kennedy, Lexinton, Mass: D C Health & Co.

Munhall, P (1982). 'Nursing philosophy and nursing research: in apposition or opposition?' *Nursing Research* 31:3 (May–June), pp. 176–177, 181.

Munhall, P L — Oiler, C J (eds) (1986). *Nursing Research: A Qualitative Perspective*. Norwalk, Conn: Appleton-Century-Crofts.

Murphy, J W (1986). 'Phenomenological social science: research in the public interest'. *The Social Science Journal* 23:3, pp. 327–343.

Natanson, M A (1973a). *Edmund Husserl: Philosopher of Infinite Tasks*. Evanston: Northwestern University Press.

Natanson, M (1973b). 'Phenomenology and the social sciences'. In *Phenomenology and the Social Sciences*, ed. M Natanson, Vol. I, Evanston: Northwestern University Press, pp. 3–44.

Natanson, M (1974). *Phenomenology, Role and Reason: Essays on the Coherence and Deformation of Social Reality*. Springfield, Ill: Charles C Thomas.

Natanson, M (1977). 'Alfred Schutz symposium: the pregivenness of sociality'. In *Interdisciplinary Phenomenology*, eds D Ihde and R M Zaner, The Hague: Martinus Nijhoff, pp. 109–123.

Natanson, M (1985). 'Descriptive phenomenology'. In *Descriptions*, eds D Ihde and H J Silverman, Albany: State University of New York Press, pp. 2–13.

Newman, M A — Moch, S D (1991). 'Life patterns of persons with coronary heart disease'. *Nursing Science Quarterly* 4:4 (Winter), pp. 161–167.

O'Connor, R (1979). 'Ortega's reformulation of Husserlian phenomenology'. *Philosophy and Phenomenological Research* 40:1 (September), pp. 53–63.

O'Hara, M (1989). 'When I use the term *Humanistic Psychology* ... ' *Journal of Humanistic Psychology* 29:2 (Spring), pp. 263–273.

O'Neill, J (1974). 'Introduction: Perception, Expression and History'. In *Phenomenology, Language and Sociology: Selected Essays of Maurice Merleau-Ponty*, ed. J O'Neill, London: Heinemann, pp. xi–lxii.

O'Neill, J (1985). 'Phenomenological sociology'. *Revue Canadienne de Sociologie et d'Anthropologie / Canadian Review of Sociology and Anthropology* 22:5 (December), pp. 748–770.

Oiler, C J (1986). 'Phenomenology: the method'. In *Nursing Research: A Qualitative Perspective* eds P L Munhall and C J Oiler, Norwalk, Conn: Appleton-Century-Crofts, pp. 69–84.

Okrent, M (1988). *Heidegger's Pragmatism: Understanding, Being, and the Critique of Metaphysics*. Ithaca, NY: Cornell University Press.

Ortega y Gasset, J (1963). *Concord and Liberty*. New York: Norton.

Omery, A (1983). 'Phenomenology: a method for nursing research'. *Advances in Nursing Science* 5:2, pp. 49–63.

Ott, H (1993). *Martin Heidegger: A Political Life*. London: HarperCollins.

Palmer, R E (1969). *Hermeneutics: Interpretation Theory in Schleiermacher, Dilthey, Heidegger, and Gadamer*. Evanston, Ill: Northwestern University Press.

Peirce, C S (1931–1958). *The Collected Papers of Charles Sanders Peirce*, Vols 1–6, eds C Hartshorne and P Weiss, Vols 7–8 eds A Burks, Cambridge, Mass: Harvard University Press.

Percy, W (1990). 'The loss of the creature'. In *Ways of Reading: An Anthology for Writers*, eds D Bartholomae and A Petrosky, 2nd edition, Boston: Bedford Books of St Martin's Press, pp. 462–476.

Peters, T (1991). *The Cosmic Self: A Penetrating Look at Today's New Age Movements*. New York: HarperCollins.

Pickles, J (1985). *Phenomenology, Science and Geography: Spatiality and the Human Sciences*. Cambridge: Cambridge University Press.

Pöggeler, O (1978). 'Being as appropriate'. In *Heidegger and Modern Philosophy: Critical Essays*, ed. M Murray, New Haven: Yale University Press, pp. 84–115.

Pöggeler, O (1991). 'Heidegger's political self-understanding'. In *The Heidegger Controversy: A Critical Reader*, ed. R Wolin, New York: Columbia University Press, pp. 198–244.

Psathas, G (1973). 'Introduction'. In *Phenomenological Sociology: Issues and Applications*, ed. G Psathas, New York: Wiley, pp. 1–21.

Psathas, G (1977). 'Ethnomethodology as a phenomenological approach in the social sciences'. In *Interdisciplinary Phenomenology*, eds D Ihde and R M Zaner, The Hague: Martinus Nijhoff, pp. 73–98.

Rather, M L (1992). '"Nursing as a way of thinking": Heideggerian hermeneutical analysis of the lived experience of the returning RN'. *Research in Nursing and Health* 15:1 (February), pp. 47–55.

Ray, M A (1985). 'A philosophical method to study nursing phenomena'. In *Qualitative Research Methods*, ed. M M Leininger, Philadelphia: Saunders, pp. 81–92.

Rehorick, D A (1991). 'Pickling human geography: the souring of phenomenology in the human sciences'. *Human Studies* 14:4 (October), pp. 359–369.

Rich, A (1990). 'When we dead awaken: writing as re-vision'. In *Ways of Reading: An Anthology for Writers*, eds D Bartholomae and A Petrosky, 2nd edition, Boston: Bedford Books of St Martin's Press, pp. 482–496.

Richardson, W (1963). *Heidegger: Through Phenomenology to Thought*. The Hague: Martinus Nijhoff.

Ricoeur, P (1967). *Husserl: An Analysis of His Phenomenology*. Evanston: Northwestern University Press.

Robinson, J C (1987). *Radical Literary Education: A Classroom Experiment with Wordsworth's 'Ode'*. Madison: University of Wisconsin Press.

Rochberg-Halton, E (1986). *Meaning and Modernity: Social Theory in the Pragmatic Attitude*. Chicago: University of Chicago Press.

Rogers, C R (1961). *On Becoming a Person: A Therapist's View of Psychotherapy*. London: Constable.

Rogers, C R (1969). 'Towards a science of the person'. In *Readings in Humanistic Psychology*, eds A J Sutich and M A Vick, New York: Macmillan, pp. 21–50.

Rogers, C R (1978). *Carl Rogers on Personal Power*. London: Constable.

Rogers, M F (1981). 'Taken-for-grantedness'. *Current Perspectives in Social Theory* 2, pp.133–151.

Rogers, M F (1983). *Sociology, Ethnomethodology, and Experience: A Phenomenological Critique*. Cambridge: Cambridge University Press.

Rorty, R (1988). 'Taking philosophy seriously'. *New Republic*, April 11, pp. 31–34.

Rose, J F (1990). 'Psychologic health of women: a phenomenologic study of women's inner strength'. *Advances in Nursing Science* 12:2 (January), pp. 56–70.

Rowan, J (1989). 'Two humanistic psychologies or one?' *Journal of Humanistic Psychology* 29:2 (Spring), pp. 224–229.

Sadler, W A (Jr) (1969). *Existence and Love: A New Approach in Existential Phenomenology*. New York: Charles Scribner's Sons.

Sallis, J (1973). *Phenomenology and the Return to Beginnings*. Pittsburgh: Duquesne University Press.

Sartre, J-P (1956a). *Being and Nothingness: An Essay on Phenomenological Ontology*. New York: Philosophical Library.

Sartre, J-P (1956b). 'Existentialism is an humanism'. In *Existentialism from Dostoevsky to Sartre*, ed. W Kaufmann, Cleveland: Meridian Books, pp. 287–311.

Schachtel, E G (1963). *Metamorphosis: On the Development of Affect, Perception, Attention and Memory*. London: Routledge & Kegan Paul.

Scheler, M (1974ff.) 'Scham und Schamgefühl'. In *Gesammelte Werke* Vol.10: *Schriften aus dem Nachlass*, eds M Scheler and M S Frings, Bern: Francke.

Schrag, C O (1967). 'Phenomenology, ontology, and history in the philosophy of Heidegger'. In *Phenomenology: The Philosophy of Edmund Husserl and Its Interpretation*, ed. J J Kockelmans, New York: Doubleday, pp. 277–293.

Schuhmann, K (1985). 'Structuring the phenomenological field: reflections on a Daubert manuscript'. In *Phenomenology in Practice and Theory*, ed. W S Hamrick, The Hague: Martinus Nijhoff, pp. 3–17.

Schutz, A (1962). *Collected Papers*. Vol. I. Ed. M Natanson. The Hague: Martinus Nijhoff.

Schutz, A (1964). *Collected Papers*. Vol. II. Ed. A Brodersen. The Hague: Martinus Nijhoff.

Schutz, A (1966). *Collected Papers*. Vol. III. Ed. I Schutz. The Hague: Martinus Nijhoff.

Schutz, A (1967). *The Phenomenology of the Social World*. Evanston: Northwestern University Press.

Schutz, A and Luckmann, T (1973). *The Structure of the Life-World*. Evanston: Northwestern University Press.

Sheehan, T (1993). 'Reading a life: Heidegger and hard times'. In *The Cambridge Companion to Heidegger*, ed. C B Guignon, Cambridge: Cambridge University Press, pp. 70–96.

Smith, Q (1978). 'Husserl's theory of the phenomenological reduction in the *Logical Investigations*'. *Philosophy and Phenomenological Research* 39:3, pp. 433–437.

Solomon, R C (1988). *Continental Philosophy since 1750: The Rise and Fall of the Self. A History of Western Philosophy*, Vol. 7. Oxford: Oxford University Press.

Spiegelberg, H (1972). *Phenomenology in Psychology and Psychiatry: A Historical Introduction*. Evanston: Northwestern University Press.

Spiegelberg, H (1975). *Doing Phenomenology: Essays on and in Phenomenology*. The Hague: Martinus Nijhoff.

Spiegelberg, H (1981a). 'Husserl's and Peirce's phenomenologies: coincidence or interaction'. In *The Context of the Phenomenological Movement*, The Hague: Martinus Nijhoff, pp. 27–50.

Spiegelberg, H (1981b). 'Husserl's approach to phenomenology for Americans: a letter and its sequel'. In *The Context of the Phenomenological Movement*, The Hague: Martinus Nijhoff, pp. 173–192.

Spiegelberg, H (1982). *The Phenomenological Movement: A Historical Introduction*. 3rd edition. Boston: Martinus-Nijhoff.

Srubar, I (1984). 'On the origin of "phenomenological" sociology'. *Human Studies* 7 (1984), pp. 163–189.

Steiner, G (1978). *Heidegger*. Hassocks, Sussex: Harvester Press.

Stikkers, K W (1985). "Phenomenology as psychic technique of non-resistance". In *Phenomenology in Practice and Theory*, ed. W S Hamrick, Dordrecht: Martinus Nijhoff, pp. 129–151.

Taylor, C (1985). *Human Agency and Language: Philosophical Papers*. Vol. 1. Cambridge: Cambridge University Press.

Taylor, C (1989). *Sources of the Self: The Making of the Modern Identity*. Cambridge, Mass: Harvard University Press.

Thévenaz, P (1962). *What is Phenomenology? and Other Essays*. Chicago: Quadrangle.

Tiryakian, E A (1962). *Sociologism and Existentialism: Two Perspectives on the Individual and Society*. Englewood Cliffs, NJ: Prentice-Hall.

Turner, J H (1986). *The Structure of Sociological Theory*. 4th edition. Chicago: Dorsey.

van Kaam, A (1966). *Existential Foundations of Psychology*. Pittsburgh: Duquesne University Press.

van Manen, M (1990). *Researching Lived Experience: Human Science for an Action Sensitive Pedagogy*. Ontario: Althouse Press.

Watson, J (1988). *Nursing: Human Science and Human Caring. A Theory of Nursing*. New York: National League for Nursing.

Watson, P (1991). 'Care or control: questions and answers for psychiatric nursing practice'. *Nursing Praxis in New Zealand* 6:2 (March), pp. 10–14.

Weber, M (1946). *From Max Weber: Essays in Sociology*. Eds H Gerth and C W Mills. New York: Oxford University Press.

Weber, M (1968). *On Charisma and Institution Building*. Ed. S N Eisenstadt. Chicago: University of Chicago Press.

Weinberg, H L (1959). *Levels of Knowing and Existence*. New York: Harper & Row.

Welte, B (1982). 'God in Heidegger's thought'. *Philosophy Today* 26 (Spring), pp. 85–100.

Whetstone, W R — Reid, J C (1991). 'Health promotion of older adults: perceived barriers'. *Journal of Advanced Nursing* 16:11 (November), pp. 1343–1349.

Wild, J (1955). *The Challenge of Existentialism*. Bloomington: Indiana University Press.

Wolf, Z R (1991). 'Nurses' experiences giving postmortem care to patients who have donated organs: a phenomenological study'. *Scholarly Inquiry for Nursing Practice: An International Journal* 5:2 (Summer), pp. 73–87.

Wolff, K H (1972). *Surrender and Catch: A Palimpsest Story*. Sorokin Lectures, No.3. Saskatoon: University of Saskatchewan Press.

Wolff, K H (1976). *Surrender and Catch: Experience and Inquiry Today*. Dordrecht: Reidel.

Wolff, K H (1983). *Beyond the Sociology of Knowledge: An Introduction and a Development*. Lanham, NY: University Press of America.

Wolff, K H (1984). 'Surrender-and-catch and phenomenology'. *Human Studies* 7:2, pp.191–210.

Wolff, K H (1989a). *O Loma! Constituting a Self (1977–1984)*. Northhampton, Mass: Hermes House.

Wolff, K H (1989b). 'From nothing to sociology'. *Philosophy of the Social Sciences* 19, pp.321–339.

Wolff, K H (1990). *Survival and Sociology: Vindicating the Human Subject*. New Brunswick, NJ: Transaction.

Wolin, R (1991). 'French Heidegger wars'. In *The Heidegger Controversy: A Critical Reader*, ed. R Wolin, New York: Columbia University Press, pp. 282–310.

Wondolowski, C and Davis, D K (1991). 'The lived experience of health in the oldest old: a phenomenological study'. *Nursing Science Quarterly* 4:3 (Fall), pp. 113–118.

Wood, F G (1991). 'The meaning of caregiving'. *Rehabilitation Nursing* 16:4 (July-August), pp.195–198.

Zaner, R M (1970). *The Way of Phenomenology: Criticism as a Philosophical Discipline*. New York: Pegasus.

Zerwekh, J V (1992). 'Laying the groundwork for family self-help: locating families, building trust, and building strength'. *Public Health Nursing* 9:1 (March), pp. 15–21.

Zimmerman, D H and Pollner, M (1971). 'The everyday world as a phenomenon'. In *Understanding Everyday Life: Toward the Reconstruction of Sociological Knowledge*, ed. J D Douglas, London: Routledge & Kegan Paul, pp. 80–103.

Index